SUPPLEMENT NO 2 TO VOLUME 76, 1998, OF THE

BULLETIN

OF THE WORLD HEALTH ORGANIZATION
DE L'ORGANISATION MONDIALE DE LA SANTE

THE SCIENTIFIC JOURNAL OF WHO • LA REVUE SCIENTIFIQUE DE L'OMS

GLOBAL DISEASE ELIMINATION AND ERADICATION AS PUBLIC HEALTH STRATEGIES

PROCEEDINGS OF A CONFERENCE HELD IN ATLANTA, GEORGIA, USA
23–25 FEBRUARY 1998

EDITED BY
R.A. GOODMAN, K.L. FOSTER,
F.L. TROWBRIDGE, & J.P. FIGUEROA

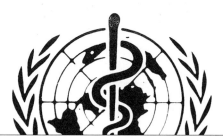

WORLD HEALTH ORGANIZATION, GENEVA • ORGANISATION MONDIALE DE LA SANTE, GENEVE

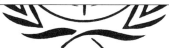

Publications of the World Health Organization enjoy copyright protection in accordance with the provisions of Protocol 2 of the Universal Copyright Convention.

For rights of reproduction or translation of WHO publications, in part or *in toto*, application should be made to the Office of Publications, World Health Organization, 1211 Geneva 27, Switzerland. The World Health Organization welcomes such applications.

The views expressed in the articles in this Supplement are those of the authors and may differ from those held by the World Health Organization.

The designations employed and the presentation of the material in this publication do not imply the expression of any opinion whatsoever on the part of the Secretariat of the World Health Organization concerning the legal status of any country, territory, city, or area or of its authorities, or concerning the delimitation of its frontiers or boundaries.

The mention of specific companies or of certain manufacturers' products does not imply that they are endorsed or recommended by the World Health Organization in preference to others of a similar nature which are not mentioned. Errors and omissions excepted, the names of proprietary products are distinguished by initial capital letters.

ISBN 92 4 068760 2
Typeset in Hong Kong
Printed in Finland
98/12135 — Best Set/Vammala — 6700

CONTENTS

PREFACE

R.A. Goodman,[1] K.L. Foster,[2] F.L. Trowbridge,[3] & J.P. Figueroa[4]

This Supplement to the *Bulletin of the World Health Organization* presents the Proceedings of the Conference on Global Disease Elimination and Eradication as Public Health Strategies, which was held in Atlanta, GA, USA, on 23–25 February 1998. The Conference was co-sponsored by WHO and many national and international agencies (see Annex C). One of the co-sponsors, the Task Force for Child Survival and Development (TFCSD), also served as the Conference Secretariat. The Conference focused on two main objectives: to evaluate the role of elimination or eradication of diseases in the context of local and global health problems and sustainable health development; and to identify the specific conditions and diseases with the highest potential for elimination and eradication. This Conference was without precedent in terms of the broad expertise and stature of the invited participants and, perhaps more importantly, its aim to examine simultaneously the categories of noninfectious conditions, infectious diseases, and health systems, all in relation to the potential for global disease elimination and eradication.

Over 200 invited persons with expertise in international health and selected diseases or health conditions participated in the Conference. These experts represented a broad range of international organizations, academic institutions, other programmes, and countries (see list of participants, Annex B). Their experiences encompassed several key disciplines, including vertically organized disease control and prevention programmes, health systems infrastructure development, basic laboratory research, epidemiology, economics, and behavioural sciences.

The goal of the Conference was to produce practical, concrete recommendations to assist governments, nongovernmental, multinational, and other organizations in their consideration of disease elimination and eradication efforts. Accordingly, the Conference was structured first to provide pertinent background information and perspectives on ongoing elimination and eradication programmes. Participants were then presented with the results of a pre-Conference survey intended to identify potential candidate noninfectious and infectious conditions. This information was used by five workgroups (sustainable health development; noninfectious conditions; and bacterial, viral, and parasitic diseases) to assist in framing their deliberations.

Because of the historical importance of the Conference, the organizers sought to produce in the Proceedings both the spirit and the substance of the meeting. The goal of the editors was to ensure an accurate record of the Conference, while retaining the uniquely diverse expression of each contributor. The published Proceedings therefore present the plenary papers reporting on the background and previous programmes, followed by papers updating ongoing disease elimination and eradication programmes. Papers addressing candidate diseases/conditions for elimination or eradication precede the conclusions and recommendations of each of the five workgroups. The workgroup reports are followed by comments made during open discussion and by a synthesis. The Annexes include detailed fact sheets about specific diseases/conditions for the use by workgroup members. The Conference summary also contains points discussed by a small workgroup, convened in Atlanta on 1–2 June 1998, to consider critical issues identified during the Conference.

Meeting the goals of the published Proceedings, one of the priority outcomes of the Conference, required an extraordinary effort by the contributors and the professional staff of TFCSD and CDC. In particular, we thank Kim Koporc and Richard Conlon for their efforts, and Dr Walter Dowdle for his unfailing support. In addition, we are grateful to Dr Ian Neil, Editor of the *Bulletin of the World Health Organization*, for his flexibility during the development of the Proceedings. Finally, we would like to add our own note of thanks in acknowledging the efforts of many others who were involved in the Conference, including the co-sponsoring organizations, the workgroup rapporteurs, the primary authors of all the other papers, the dedicated staff of TFCSD for their support in facilitating the Conference, Dr Rob Lyerla of CDC, and the experts who developed the fact sheets. The contributions of all these persons and organizations ensured the success of the Conference and the timely development of these Proceedings and should assist in promoting health through the control, elimination, and eradication of disease.

[1] Editor in Chief (Financial Management Office, Centers for Disease Control and Prevention, Atlanta, GA, USA).
[2] Associate Editor (Epidemiology Program Office, Centers for Disease Control and Prevention, Atlanta, GA, USA).
[3] Senior Editor (Executive Director, Nutrition and Health Promotion Program, International Life Sciences Institute, Atlanta, GA, USA).
[4] Senior Editor (Chief Medical Officer, Ministry of Health, Kingston, Jamaica).

ACKNOWLEDGEMENTS

The Conference on Global Disease Elimination and Eradication as Public Health Strategies was the result of the efforts of many individuals, participating organizations, and co-sponsors. The Conference Secretariat, which coordinated the meeting, acknowledges the hard work of the members of the programme planning and arrangements committees, the authors of the fact sheets, and the scientific advisors. We are grateful to the Conference Moderators and Co-Chairs, and to Dr Peter Bell, Dr Nat Bhamarapravati, Dr David Brandling-Bennett, Dr Claire Broome, Dr Denis Broun, Dr Suriadi Gunawan, Dr Mamoun Homeida, Dr Festo Kavishe, Dr Helena Makela, Dr Edward Mbidde, Dr P.R. Narayanan, Dr Peter Ndumbe Jamie Sepulveda and Dr Kean Wang — all of whom helped to keep the Conference on time and on track. We extend our special thanks to the cosponsors of the Conference (listed in Annex C), without whose support and generosity the meeting could not have been held. Although it is not possible to list the names of all the many persons who played critical roles in the success of the Conference, a few deserve special recognition. These include Richard Conlon for his operational skills, creativity, and resourcefulness, and the following members of the Secretariat staff: Corey Anderson, Cheryl Bauerle, Regina Cannon, Amy Gray, Kim Koporc, Karen Lindauer, Pat Richmond, Sara Stefero and Carol Walters, and the graduate student volunteers from Emory University. Finally, we thank Dr Rick Goodman for serving as Editor in Chief of the Proceedings, and for his enthusiastic support, insight, and tireless dedication to the success of the Conference.

Walter R. Dowdle, on behalf of the Task Force
for Child Survival and Development,
Conference Secretariat

ACRONYMS

AFB	acid-fast bacilli
AFP	acute flaccid paralysis
AIDS	acquired immunodeficiency syndrome
APOC	African Programme for Onchocerciasis Control
AUSAID	Australian Agency for International Development
BASICS	Basic Support for Institutionalizing Child Survival
BCG	bacille Calmette–Guérin
CD	Chagas disease
CDC	Centers for Disease Control and Prevention
CIDA	Canadian International Development Agency
CLD	chronic liver disease
CRS	congenital rubella syndrome
CTD	Control of Tropical Diseases programme
DALDs	disability-adjusted life days
DALYs	disability-adjusted life years
DANIDA	Danish International Development Agency
DEC	diethylcarbamazine
DEP	Drancunculiasis Eradication Programme
DFID	Department for International Development, United Kingdom
DNA	deoxyribonucleic acid
DOTS	directly observed treatment, short course
DPT	diphtheria–pertussis–tetanus vaccine
DPT3	three doses of DPT vaccine
EDTA	ethylenediaminetetraacetic acid
EP	elimination/eradication programmes
EPI	Expanded Programme on Immunization
ERR	estimated rate of return
FADNTDs	folic-acid-dependent neural tube defects
GDP	gross domestic product
GIS	Geographical Information Systems
HALYs	handicap-adjusted life years
HAV	hepatitis A virus
HBV	hepatitis B virus
Hib	*Haemophilus influenzae* type B
HIS	health information systems
HIV	human immunodeficiency virus
ICCs	interagency coordination committees
ID	iron deficiency
IDA	iron-deficiency anaemia
IDD	iodine-deficiency disease
IEC	Information, education, communication
ILO	International Labour Organization
ILSI	International Life Sciences Institute
IPV	inactivated poliovirus
IUMS	International Union of Microbiological Societies
JICA	Japan International Cooperation Agency
KAP	knowledge, attitude, practices
KEMRI	Kenya Medical Research Institute
LGA	local government area
MCH	maternal and child health
MDT	multiple drug therapy
MECACAR	international polio effort by 18 countries in the Middle East, Caucasus, and Central Asian Republics
MOH	Ministry of Health
MSG	monosodium glutamate
NCIH	National Council for International Health
NGO	nongovernmental organization
NGDO	nongovernmental development organization
NIAID	National Institute of Allergy and Infectious Diseases
NIDs	national immunization days
NIH	National Institutes of Health
NIS	Newly Independent States of the former USSR
NT	neonatal tetanus
OCP	Onchocerciasis Control Programme
OEPA	Onchocerciasis Elimination Program for the Americas
OPV	oral poliovirus vaccine
PAHO	Pan American Health Organization
PCR	polymerase chain reaction
PEM	protein–energy malnutrition
PHC	primary health care
PHC	primary hepatocellular carcinoma
PHS	Public Health Service
PPD	purified protein derivative
RNA	ribonucleic acid
SSPE	subacute sclerosing panencephalitis
STD	sexually transmitted disease
TB	tuberculosis
TFCSD	Task Force for Child Survival and Development
TSH	thyroid-stimulating hormone

TT	tetanus toxoid	USD	United States dollar
UC	University of California	USI	universal salt iodization
UNAIDS	United Nations Programme on HIV/AIDS	VAD	vitamin A deficiency
		VVM	vaccine vial monitor
UNDP	United Nations Development Programme	WFPHA	World Federation of Public Health Associations
UNICEF	United Nations Children's Fund	WHO	World Health Organization
USAID	United States Agency for International Development	YF	yellow fever

SUMMARY

Maximum control of disease and improvement of health are the goals of every effective public health programme, whether stated or not. Each successful milestone in the reduction of a disease, each new tool for diagnosis and prevention, and each refinement in control strategy allows the establishment of new and more demanding objectives along the path to achieving these goals. Smallpox was eradicated two decades ago, and today programmes are under way to eradicate poliomyelitis and dracunculiasis (guinea-worm disease). The malaria, yellow fever, and yaws programmes in the past failed to achieve eradication, but were associated with appreciable health benefits to many and contributed to a better understanding of the biological, social, political, and economic complexities associated with disease eradication.

Achieving the ultimate goal of disease eradication has been the focus of numerous conferences, symposia, workshops, planning sessions, and public health actions for more than a century. The most recent, the 1997 Dahlem Workshop on the Eradication of Infectious Diseases, addressed the science of disease eradication. The Conference on Global Disease Elimination and Eradication as Public Health Strategies extended the Dahlem Workshop findings to consider specific infectious and noninfectious diseases and conditions in the context of sustainable health development and global priorities.

The Conference brought together over 200 participants from 81 organizations and 34 countries. It provided an unprecedented forum for the exchange of ideas among persons with different training, experience, organizational responsibilities, and points of view, each one aiming at the same goal and contributing in some way to reducing the global burden of disease. Participants from local, national, and global levels brought to the Conference a wealth of experiences that encompassed disease control and prevention programmes, health systems infrastructure development, laboratory research, epidemiology, economics, and the behavioural sciences. The Conference considered five major areas: sustainable health development; noninfectious diseases; and bacterial, parasitic, and viral diseases. Key findings and critical issues that emerged during the Conference are summarized below in relation to these five areas.

Sustainable health development

There are intrinsic and unavoidable tensions between the concepts of eradication and sustainable health development. These tensions arise because of polarization between specific rather than comprehensive goals, and a time-limited rather than long-term agenda. Acknowledging, accepting, and overcoming these tensions are essential if full advantage is to be taken of what each programme can contribute to the achievement of public health goals.

Eradication programmes should have two objectives: eradication of the disease; and strengthening and further development of health systems. Potential benefits for health development should be identified and delineated at the start of any eradication initiative. Measurable targets for achieving the development benefits should be set and the eradication programme held accountable for their realization. Resources for eradication activities should be supplementary to those available for basic health care services. Care must be taken that programmes do not divert resources from basic health services, health development, and other priorities.

Successful eradication programmes are powerful examples of effective management and should incorporate efforts to design programme activities that enhance leadership development and managerial skills which can be carried to other health programmes. Eradication programmes also should aid in the development and implementation of surveillance systems that can be readily adapted to other national priority programmes after eradication has been achieved. Finally, coordination of the development and implementation of eradication efforts with primary care services can produce biological complementarity (e.g. improvement in nutritional status, which may enhance immune responsiveness and resistance to some infectious diseases).

Noninfectious diseases

The Conference concluded that better control was achievable for certain micronutrient deficiencies (iodine, vitamin A, iron, and folic acid), lead intoxication, and silicosis, even though none of these conditions meets the requirements for eradication. Recommendations were made for reducing protein–energy malnutrition and lead intoxication and for accelerating the attainment of global goals for the control of micronutrient deficiencies. Micronutrient supplementation should be enhanced by taking advantage of food fortification and the opportunities presented by the existing health infrastructure and immunization programmes.

Bacterial diseases

Congenital syphilis, trachoma, and *Haemophilus influenzae* type b (Hib) infection in some countries are candidates for elimination, but no bacterial diseases were judged to be current candidates for eradication. The WHO neonatal tetanus "elimination goal" of <1 case per 1000 live births in every district was considered laudable and attainable. Eradication was considered to be a long-term goal for tuberculosis and Hib infection. Bacterial diseases represent a major disease burden and have substantial research needs before eradication goals can be established. Aggressive action was strongly recommended to improve global control of bacterial conditions.

Parasitic diseases

Dracunculiasis (guinea-worm disease) eradication is in progress. Although no additional parasitic diseases were considered to be current candidates for eradication, the increasing availability of potent, long-acting drugs brings extraordinary opportunities for overcoming onchocerciasis and lymphatic filariasis, and the effectiveness of the strategy for controlling the triatomid vectors provides similar opportunities for American trypanosomiasis (Chagas disease). The workgroup concluded that onchocerciasis (river blindness) and lymphatic filariasis (caused by all *Wuchereria* and most *Brugia* infections) could be eliminated and possibly eradicated in the future. For the 5% of cases of lymphatic filariasis caused by *Brugia malayi*, which also has an animal reservoir (in South-east Asia), elimination of disease, but not infection, is feasible. Similarly, for Chagas disease where animal reservoirs exist, elimination of disease, but not infection, is feasible.

Viral diseases

Poliomyelitis eradication is in progress. Measles and rubella were concluded to be possible candidates for eradication within the next 10–15 years. Measles transmission appears to have been interrupted for various periods in many countries in the Americas; elimination has not yet been demonstrated in other regional settings. The workgroup recommended that developed countries should proceed with elimination of measles as a step towards eradication. In other countries, accelerating measles control should be the priority, especially in areas with high mortality. Developing countries should proceed cautiously to more costly measles elimination programmes to avoid undermining the poliomyelitis eradication

effort. Experience gained from regional and country interventions should be used to refine the strategies for eventual eradication.

The eradication of rubella as an add-on to measles eradication was felt to be biologically plausible. However, several issues first need to be addressed, including the burden of rubella disease (human and financial), the marginal cost of adding rubella to a measles eradication effort, and demonstration that elimination is programmatically feasible and sustainable in a large geographical area.

The workgroup urged stronger international efforts to control rabies, yellow fever, and Japanese encephalitis by using existing measures, but none of these diseases was considered suitable as a candidate for eradication because of the existence of a nonhuman reservoir. Viral hepatitis A eradication was concluded to be biologically feasible but further demonstration of sustainable elimination was first required.

Viral hepatitis B was not considered to be a current candidate for eradication because of the multi-generation programme necessary to overcome the effect of long-term virus persistence. However, the workgroup recommended immunization in all countries to maximize the likelihood of eliminating transmission of hepatitis B virus.

Conclusion

The Conference provided a multidisciplinary forum for addressing issues related to disease elimination and eradication and their relationship to sustainable development in health. There was widespread agreement that an eradication programme could have many positive effects on health systems development and that explicit efforts should be made to maximize these positive effects as well as minimize any negative effects. Community mobilization and organization should be seen as a component of sustainable health development, with the additional potential for disease control and eradication. Poliomyelitis and dracunculiasis eradication efforts are already under way. Measles and rubella are possible candidates for eradication. Congenital syphilis, trachoma, and Hib infection are candidates for elimination in some countries. River blindness (onchocerciasis) and lymphatic filariasis (*W. bancrofti*) could be eliminated and possibly eradicated at some time in the future.

Discussions in the final plenary session centred on concerns about the misuse and misunderstanding of the term elimination, since this term is often not clearly distinguished from eradication. Also addressed was the need to bring the findings of the

Conference to other forums to expand discussion of international health goals and strengthen the mutual ties between sustainable health development and disease control and eradication efforts. Finally, the Conference suggested that a small group convene to further address the topic of definitions and to identify next steps for disseminating and implementing the recommendations of the Conference (see report on p. 113).

CONTEXT OF DISEASE ELIMINATION AND ERADICATION

Keynote address

Ralph H. Henderson[1]

Good Morning! We can look forward to an exciting week and, more importantly, through our deliberations and debates, to making contributions to public policy and political action which will improve the effectiveness of public health programmes. That is obviously a tall order, but certainly not out of proportion to the stature of this audience. The World Health Organization and the Pan American Health Organization are pleased to be sponsors of this conference and are glad to join with the many other sponsors who are such distinguished actors in the arena of public health.

I will not try to keep you in suspense about whether or not I think disease elimination and eradication are potentially effective public health strategies, in case any of you were wondering. I think they certainly can be effective. And while I think they have a number of especially attractive attributes as strategies, I see them as part of a continuum of strategies bounded on one side by global disease eradication — that is, zero cases and zero risk of cases, and on the other by disease control — that is, a reduction in cases by some defined amount. Intermediary strategies would include disease elimination (zero cases but with continuing risk) and our famous WHO term, elimination of the disease as a public health problem (reduction of cases below what is considered to be a public health risk).

So, given my general support, I would like to direct my remarks to some aspects of these strategies which can be summarized by three quotations:

(1) *For if the trumpet give an uncertain sound, who shall prepare himself to the battle?* (1 Corinthians: 14.8).

(2) *He who would do good must do it in minute particulars; general good is the plea of the scoundrel, hypocrite and flatterer.* (William Blake).

(3) *The fox knows many things, but the hedgehog knows one big thing.* (Archilochus).

For the first quote, I am indebted to Bill Foege, who called my attention to *Certain Trumpets: the nature of leadership*, a book by Gary Wills (New York, Simon & Schuster, 1994). Because leaders do not act in isolation, the book is also one about man-

agement, typically the management of attaining, or trying to attain, some great cause. And disease elimination and eradication are certainly great causes. Few would argue that we can achieve disease elimination or eradication with an "uncertain" trumpet. We need a clear call, and constituencies willing and able to heed it.

It was from Professor David Bradley of the London School of Tropical Medicine and Hygiene that I first heard the quote from William Blake that "He who would do good must do it in minute particulars . . .". And I find myself using it frequently, often in debates relating to such broad aspirations as the elimination of poverty, the prevention of violence, and even the attainment of "health for all". For, to be achieved, these aspirations must be dissected until one identifies specifically what can and must be done, the "minute particular" forming the building block of the larger cause. As a former colleague and friend used to say: "If you are going to eat a buffalo, do it one bite at a time."

Yet the act of blowing a "certain trumpet" for a "minute particular" sometimes leads some people, if not always the multitudes, to believe that the trumpet blower (like the hedgehog) only knows one thing, and does not (like the fox) know the many things that put each action into an appropriate overall context. That quote comes from the Greek poet Archilocus. A more modern quote comes from Lotfi Zadeh, the father of "fuzzy logic", who said "When the only tool you know is a hammer, everything begins to look like a nail."

This leads me to one aspect of our week's deliberations. When we choose a particular elimination or eradication goal, do we do so with the narrow understanding of the hedgehog or with the broader vision of the fox? Do we judiciously choose elimination or eradication because it is the best strategy or only because it is, like the hammer, the only tool we know? Even with a broad vision and judicious choice, however, circumstances inevitably arise in which one is unable to achieve an essential elimination or eradication objective without compromising a broader health services development goal. So part of our discussions will need to address what may or may not be appropriate trade-offs between the two, including the possible negative consequences of failure of a specific elimination or eradication initiative.

In his book, Gary Wills argues that, important as good leadership is, the *goal selected* and the *fol-*

[1] Assistant Director-General, World Health Organization, 1211 Geneva 27, Switzerland.

lowers are also essential for success and that the initiative in question must be right for the *historical moment*. Without quarrelling about these elements, I would like to argue that our "historical moment" is favouring a different kind of leadership than the examples described by Wills. What is that historical moment? I see it being characterized as a series of "-izations". They are, among others, global*ization*, decentral*ization*, democrat*ization* and privat*ization*. One result of these is a world in which there are more and more people and organizations involved in more and more aspects of life in all countries of the world.

In the "for-profit" sector, a result of these "-izations", or at least a desired result, is more competition. While this is generally regarded as a positive benefit for society as a whole by encouraging the more efficient use of resources, there is concern that such efficiency is eroding equity and widening the gaps in incomes and health between the rich and the poor and that it is leading to the increased promotion of unhealthy products, a notable example being tobacco in developing countries. In the public sector, however, it seems to me that these "-izations" emphasize the need for cooperation rather than competition. The cooperation of the increasing number of "stake-holders" involved in sectors such as health or education cannot be commanded or forced through economic pressures; it must be solicited. And more and more of these stake-holders are leaders in their own right. They have their own powerful trumpets.

So the public sector leader of today has the primary task of harmonizing many trumpets. The more resources that are required, the more the various trumpet players need to be empowered as partners in the endeavour. And the more the focus of all partners needs to be on outcomes rather than inputs. They must be able to rejoice in the *results* and be able to forego personal or organizational recognition for their efforts, if this is what is required for success. The best leadership then becomes that which is self-effacing and which ensures that the other partners get the credit they require to keep them and their various constituencies committed. This is the kind of leadership which was described some 200 years before Christ in the *Tao Te Ching*:

"A leader is best
When people barely know he exists.
Of a good leader, who talks little,
When his work is done, his aim fulfilled,
They will say, "We did this ourselves."

The choice of highly specific goals is essential for success in such a "multi-leader" or "multi-partner" context. They must have two special fea-tures. First, they must be easily measurable in easily understood terms. This permits all partners to obtain clear feedback on progress and on their own participation in the effort. The broader the partnership, the more important that measurability and feedback become. Second, these goals must be narrow; they must be "minute particulars". This facilitates the measurement and feedback problem, but it is also important in achieving the type of consensus needed to make broad partnerships work. I suppose this is a paradox, as it would seem more logical that broad goals, e.g. the eradication of poverty, would be the most effective in achieving broad partnerships. But I think such partnerships have a high risk of being illusions.

A broad goal often simply permits the so-called partners to continue "business as usual", claiming they are an essential part of the overall effort whether or not they really are. A narrow goal may attract fewer partners, but those partners who are attracted are forced to confront the specifics of what they are being asked to do, and can be held accountable for their commitments. When the specific input needs are clearly defined, "turf" battles are minimized, as most partners easily see in what way they can best contribute — where their particular comparative advantages shine. I champion the narrow goal as a more effective means of forging real consensus and collaboration than the broad goal. These characteristics of goals are, of course, generic to good management in any field, but are especially important in managing enterprises that rely on "multi-leader" coalitions. I cannot think of any goals that fit these characteristics better than disease elimination or eradication goals. This gives them a special utility in serving as rallying-points for coalitions of interested partners. This, in turn, helps to ensure that these goals can receive the support required to attain them.

There is another feature of disease elimination or eradication goals which makes them especially attractive: they bring direct and immediate benefits to those at risk of the diseases in question. By and large, those most at risk are those most socially and economically vulnerable. So the immediate benefits often go, not simply to the poor, but to the poorest of the poor. And they extend to all future generations as well, poor and rich.

In resource mobilization, of course, we do argue for support based on the benefits returned to the contributors. We will hear more in this meeting about the benefits to broader health systems which disease elimination and eradication initiatives can bring, and more about how sustained health benefits provide a powerful stimulus to broader social and economic development. Yet I have to confess that I think there is another major motivation for many partners engaged in disease elimination or eradication. It is simply the opportunity to achieve any concrete benefit whatsoever in the short-term! This is quite a rare event in international development.

Most of you are well aware of what a good example of multi-partner leadership is being provided by the eradication of poliomyelitis. Rotary International is one of the primary partners. Rotary's vision and goal have now become institutionalized and are being passionately supported by thousands of Rotary Clubs and by tens of thousands, if not hundreds of thousands, of individual Rotarians. Many seem only marginally aware that there are other major partners involved and have taken upon themselves the challenge of ensuring success! And the leadership they are exerting, from community to national to global level, is proving absolutely critical to that success.

Rotary is certainly not the only "polio partner", as most of you know well. Leadership is also coming from a broad array of others: from nongovernmental organizations, from national governments, from national institutions such as CDC and NIH, from international development agencies such as USAID, from the World Bank, the Inter-American Development Bank and the other Regional Banks, from other members of the United Nations family, including WHO and UNICEF, and from the private sector. This multiple-leadership pattern is also typical of our other initiatives, including guinea-worm disease eradication and the elimination of leprosy, onchocerciasis and lymphatic filariasis.

Yet, if poliomyelitis and several other diseases, which we will be considering, do provide us with attractive models of disease elimination and eradication which can be used as effective public health strategies, I think the Conference organizers may also be asking a further question. I interpret this as being whether disease elimination or eradication goals are so potentially powerful as rallying points for social action that one should intentionally search out candidate-diseases as an explicit mobilization strategy. In other words, might one intentionally single out a disease for elimination or eradication primarily because of its social-mobilization and more general development benefits rather than because of its more narrowly defined disease-reduction benefits? A related question, posed by one of our colleagues at this meeting, is whether an elimination/eradication orientation might not also imply giving priority to developing the tools required for elimination or eradication over tools that might be adequate for simple control.

While I think some caution in embracing a pervasive elimination/eradication orientation is warranted, I see the example of Jim Grant of UNICEF and his success in promoting narrow goals as an explicit strategy for social mobilization and broad development aims as a powerful argument for pursuing broad goals through narrow actions. He insisted that the key to mobilizing political leaders is to give them "do-able", if ambitious, packages to implement. Of course, Jim did not, in fact, primarily promote disease elimination or eradication, although he was certainly a member of the club with his support for the elimination of micronutrient deficiencies and for the eradication of poliomyelitis. His main focus, however, was on other areas where it seemed that rapid progress should be possible, such as growth monitoring, oral rehydration, breast-feeding and immunization. So, although disease elimination and eradication do provide quite special opportunities, they are certainly not the only "minute particulars" which can be elements of effective public health strategies.

I would like to conclude by summarizing my arguments. Leaders and "certain trumpets" are needed for success. Our "historical moment", however, is one in which many command certain, and often very loud, trumpets. The successful leader, and especially the successful public sector leader, is one who can persuade these various trumpet players to join in harmony to support a worthy goal. This requires that the players be empowered and be given credit for their contributions. This requires, in turn, that the leader or leaders involved be more orchestra leaders, intent on the results, than themselves trumpet-blowers. Such leadership is facilitated when the goal to be attained is easily understood, when progress is easily measurable, and when the goal itself is narrow — a "minute particular". Disease elimination and eradication goals are especially effective in providing rallying points for coalitions of interested parties, although they are by no means the only rallying points. Finally, for maximum development benefits, support for "do-able", narrow goals must be obtained with the wisdom of the fox, as Jim Grant did, and not the narrow vision of the hedgehog.

Eleanor Roosevelt said: "*The future belongs to those who believe in the beauty of their dreams.*" I am sure that if she were here with us today, she would agree that those who dream of disease elimination or eradication have a special claim on that future.

Eradication: lessons from the past

Donald A. Henderson[1]

The declaration in 1980 that smallpox had been eradicated reawakened interest in disease eradication as a public health strategy. The smallpox programme's success derived, in part, from lessons learned from the preceding costly failure of the malaria eradication campaign. In turn, the smallpox programme offered important lessons with respect to other prospective disease control programmes, and these have been effectively applied in the two current global eradication initiatives, those against poliomyelitis and dracunculiasis. Taking this theme a step further, there are those who would now focus on the development of an inventory of diseases which might, one by one, be targeted either for eradication or elimination. This approach, while interesting, fails to recognize many of the important lessons learned and their broad implications for contemporary disease control programmes worldwide.

On 8 May 1980, the Thirty-third World Health Assembly declared that smallpox had been eradicated globally (1). For the first time in history, mankind had vanquished a disease. It must be borne in mind, however, that this was not the first attempt at global disease eradication but the fifth. Within a month, the Fogarty International Center convened a two-day meeting to explore the question of what diseases should be eradicated next (2). This was the first of a series of conferences of which the present one is the latest. At that first meeting, the list of diseases and conditions nominated ranged from urban rabies to periodontal disease to leprosy. Some spoke of eradication, others of elimination, and yet others of the elimination of a disease as a public health problem — however that might be defined. A tumultuous discussion eventually culminated in the decision that measles, poliomyelitis and yaws were clearly suitable for at least regional eradication but that there were many other possible candidates.

One sceptical note was made at the symposium by the two introductory speakers — Fenner & Henderson (3, 4). They reflected on the broader applicability of disease eradication from their vantage point of nearly 15 years of participation in the just concluded smallpox eradication campaign. Their basic conclusion, in brief, was that there was at that time no other suitable candidate for eradication. As they pointed out, smallpox had a number of highly favourable characteristics which facilitated eradication including the very heat-stable vaccine which protected with a single dose. No other disease came close to matching these advantages. Despite this, eradication was achieved by only the narrowest of margins. Its progress in many parts of the world and

at different times wavered between success and disaster, often only to be decided by quixotic circumstance or extraordinary performances by field staff. Nor was support for the programme generous, whatever the favourable cost–benefit ratios may have been. A number of endemic countries were themselves persuaded only with difficulty to participate in the programme; the industrialized countries were reluctant contributors; and, UNICEF, so helpful to the prior malaria programme, decided that it wanted nothing to do with another eradication programme and stated that it would make no contributions (1). Several countries did make donations of vaccine and the West African programme, directed by the US Communicable Disease Center was a critical addition. However, cash donations to WHO during the first 7 years of the smallpox programme, 1967–73, amounted to exactly US$ 79 500 (5). That is not per year but the total for that entire period.

Moreover, in 1980, support for any new eradication effort seemed especially unlikely since the smallpox eradication programme was then being critically maligned by traditional international health planners. To them, the smallpox campaign epitomized the worst of what they characterized as anachronistic, authoritarian, "top-down" programmes which they saw as anathema to the new "health for all" primary health care initiative (6).

Given these considerations, it seemed in 1980 to be little more than an interesting academic exercise to debate what next to eradicate. Having offered this view, Henderson was not again invited to the subsequent workshops, task forces, conferences and special committees on eradication which were later convened. Thus, in reflecting on the lessons to be learned from the yaws, malaria and smallpox campaigns, as I was requested to do, I come to the subject afresh and have had the opportunity to reconsider the question of the next steps in

[1] University Distinguished Service Professor, Johns Hopkins University, Baltimore, MD, USA.

eradication, based on a further 17 years of perspective.

As a reminder, the yaws and malaria campaigns began more or less at the same time, about 1955 (7, 8), and were effectively terminated some 15 years later, in 1970 or soon thereafter. The launch of each was triggered by the introduction of a new technology — an injectable single-dose long-acting penicillin, for the treatment of yaws, and the availability of large quantities of the inexpensive insecticide DDT, for use in the malaria programme. Surprisingly, prior to the launch, neither campaign could draw on the experience of large-scale pilot programmes in critical areas which would have served to demonstrate the feasibility of eradication, given the tools and resources available. If they had, neither programme would have been initiated. The existence of such prior experience would seem to be axiomatic before deciding on any eradication initiative. Yet, even the Dahlem Conference's otherwise commendable review of lessons provided by past eradication programmes effectively overlooks this fundamental precept (9).

Of the two programmes, malaria was, by far, the most important and during its 15 years of existence, it accounted for more than one-third of WHO's total expenditures and its 500-person WHO staff dwarfed all other programmes. The USA alone contributed nearly a thousand million dollars to the effort (10). The yaws campaign, in contrast, was much more modest, was little publicized, and was little known.

The strategy of the yaws programme called for the screening of patients for clinical disease and their treatment with penicillin. In all, some 160 million persons were examined and 50 million were treated in 46 countries. Besides having failed to validate the strategy in pilot studies, the programme had two glaring deficiencies. First was the fact that, for the first 10 years of its history, there was no surveillance and so it was not clear as to what was actually happening. When sample serological surveys were eventually conducted, it was discovered immediately that subclinical infections were far more prevalent than had been recognized, making eradication quite impossible. Second, there was no programme of research and thus no operational studies which might have demonstrated far earlier the futility of this exercise.

Unlike the little known yaws programme, the malaria campaign, during its existence, dominated the international health agenda (11–13). This programme was active in many countries in Latin America and South Asia as well as Ethiopia, and consumed a substantial proportion of national health expenditures as well as major inputs from WHO and USAID. The programme failed, but lessons derived

from malaria eradication were central in shaping the smallpox eradication strategy. Three operating principles were of particular importance. First was the relationship of the programme itself to the health services. It was a tenet of the malaria eradication directorate that the programme could not be successful unless it had full support from the highest level of government. This translated into a demand that the director of the programme in each country report directly to the head of government and that the malaria service function as an independent, autonomous entity with its own personnel and its own pay scales. Involvement of the community at large or of persons at the community level was not part of the overall strategy.

Second, all malaria programmes were obliged to adhere rigidly to a highly detailed, standard manual of operations. It mandated, for example, identical job descriptions in every country and even prescribed specific charts to be displayed on each office wall at each administrative level. The programme was conceived and executed as a military operation to be conducted in an identical manner whatever the battlefield. Third, the premise of the programme was that the needed technology was available and that success depended solely on meticulous attention to administrative detail in implementing the effort. Accordingly, research was considered unnecessary and was effectively suspended from the launch of the programme.

The smallpox eradication campaign had to function differently. Segregating it as an autonomous entity reporting to the head of state was neither politically acceptable nor financially feasible. With a programme budget of only US$ 2.4 million per year, there was no hope of underwriting more than a small proportion of personnel and programme costs. The programme necessarily had to function within existing health service structures and had to take advantage of available resources. This, in fact, proved advantageous, as contrary to commonly held belief, underutilized health personnel were abundant in most countries. With motivation and direction, most performed well. It was also discovered that those in the community such as teachers, religious leaders and village elders, could and did make invaluable contributions. Rigid manuals of operations intuitively made little sense given the diverse nature of national health structures and so broad goals with provision for flexibility in achieving them became the accepted mode.

Finally, research initiatives were encouraged at every level. This occurred despite the opposition of senior WHO leadership who insisted that the tools were in hand and the epidemiology was sufficiently well understood and that better management was all that was necessary to eradicate smallpox. Research initiatives included the development of new vaccination devices to replace traditional lancets; field studies, which revealed the epidemiology of the disease to be different from that described in the textbooks and, in consequence, the need for modification of basic operations; the discovery that the duration of vaccine efficacy was far longer than that normally stated, making revaccination much less important; operational research, which facilitated more efficient vaccine delivery and case detection; and studies which demonstrated conclusively that there was no animal reservoir. The principle was to ask again and again, how could this programme be made to operate more efficiently, more effectively. And, indeed, without the fruits of these research efforts, it is highly unlikely that eradication would have succeeded. Even as the last cases were being discovered, a joint Dutch–Indonesian study of a new tissue-culture vaccine was just being completed (14, 15). We hoped we would not require it, but we were prepared, should it be needed.

From the beginning of the programme, surveillance for smallpox cases was a basic strategy of the campaign. As expected, it proved to be the ultimate quality control measure, the guide to improved operations, and the yardstick of progress. These principles for conduct of an eradication programme remain valid today and, as applied in guinea-worm eradication (16) and in poliomyelitis eradication in the Americas (17) and western Asia, have proved eminently successful.

One might imagine that the subject of which diseases might next be eradicated would have been a primary topic of conversation among the large and talented group of epidemiologists who, through the late 1970s, were engaged in eradicating smallpox. In fact, I can't recall the question ever having been seriously raised or discussed. Actually, the question didn't seem especially relevant. This is not to say that we regarded the eradication of smallpox as an end in itself. Far from it.

At the time the smallpox eradication programme began, only two vaccines — BCG and smallpox — were at all widely used throughout the developing world. Few countries had organized national vaccination programmes and those that did, seldom extended much beyond the larger towns and cities; substandard and/or poorly preserved vaccines were in common use; information about disease incidence was woefully inadequate, and effective supervision was generally poor to nil.

Conceptually, as we envisaged it, an effective campaign required the development of a management structure extending from the capital city to the furthest villages; it required that mechanisms be es-

tablished to assure that fully potent and stable vaccine was used; and that plans be implemented within the existing health service structure to assure its distribution throughout the country to reach at least 80% of the inhabitants. It demanded that a national surveillance system be established, which was at that time an unknown entity in most countries; and it required that planning be done and goals established to reach a finite end-point within a given period. Most national health ministries had never before attempted an effort of this type. It seemed to us that a successful programme would provide valuable training and experience for health service staff and, most important, would create a skeleton framework permitting other activities to be added. Additional vaccines were obviously a logical further step.

In some countries, the simultaneous vaccination with two antigens began soon after the beginning of the programme. In the 20 countries of western and central Africa assisted by CDC, all countries administered smallpox and measles vaccines; in a number of countries of eastern Africa, BCG and smallpox vaccine began to be administered at the same time; and in some countries at special risk, yellow fever vaccine was also added. Few developing countries, however, provided DPT, measles or poliovirus vaccine.

With expansion of the immunization programme in mind, WHO organized, in 1970, an international meeting to review the status of vaccination internationally and to recommend model programmes (18). Recommended for general use in the developing countries were smallpox, BCG, DPT, measles and typhoid vaccines. Yellow fever and poliovirus vaccines were recommended for use but only under special circumstances. At that time, poliovirus vaccine was not generally recommended because of uncertainty as to how serious a problem poliomyelitis really was for most developing countries and because of doubts as to how efficacious poliovirus vaccine would prove to be in tropical areas. In 1974, this expanded programme of immunization was approved by the World Health Assembly; in 1977, programme leadership was strengthened and the programme began to grow (19). By then, typhoid vaccine had been dropped from the recommended list and poliovirus vaccine was added.

From the eradication of smallpox from 31 endemic countries to the implementation of effective immunization programmes for six diseases in more than 100 countries represents an enormous increase in programme complexity. Nevertheless, remarkable progress has been made in expanding and intensifying immunization activities throughout the world. In 1990, this culminated in the World Summit for Children and the nominal achievement of the goal of vaccinating 80% of the world's children against six major diseases.

One component of that programme which lagged significantly was surveillance. Not all the EPI diseases lend themselves readily to national surveillance but this did appear feasible, at least for neonatal tetanus, poliomyelitis and measles. However, persuading governments and health workers, whether national or international, that surveillance is as vital for disease control as for eradication proved to be a formidable task. In fact, until 1985, little progress was made.

At that time, Ciro de Quadros, Director of PAHO's EPI Program, visualized an approach to spur the development of national surveillance programmes in Latin America. The goal was the eradication of poliomyelitis from the Western Hemisphere. With poliomyelitis eradication having been determined to be technically feasible and, in the Americas, practicable as well, the countries of PAHO endorsed the eradication goal and, in so doing, committed themselves to the development of a hemisphere-wide surveillance effort (17). Sites reporting suspect cases each week increased from some 500 to more than 20 000. Reporting for acute flaccid paralysis was soon extended to include neonatal tetanus, measles and cholera.

During the course of poliomyelitis eradication in the Americas, new paradigms for community involvement in public health emerged as well as approaches for bringing together public and private sector agencies; national immunization days were demonstrated to be a practicable, often more efficient means for vaccine delivery; new approaches were evolved for the planning and integration of international assistance; a hemisphere-wide laboratory network was created; and new mechanisms for vaccine purchase, utilizing PAHO and UNICEF administrative channels, were established. Poliomyelitis eradication was the visible target of the programme but the agenda was far broader than this and the accomplishments likewise.

With this further background of experience, what now might I offer as lessons to the future? In contemplating this question, it is important to bear in mind that there are two diseases and only two diseases which the World Health Assembly has committed itself to eradicate — guinea-worm disease and poliomyelitis. Guinea-worm eradication, with Don Hopkins as its brilliant and persuasive advocate and strategist, has been conducted with all due attention to surveillance, to community participation, to political commitment, and to research in shaping an evolving agenda. Despite this, it lags behind scheduled targets and it is clear that its successful conclusion will require a high degree of commitment and

political skill. The outcome is not a foregone conclusion but I believe it can and will succeed.

Poliomyelitis programmes have scarcely begun in those areas of Africa and south Asia which all but thwarted global smallpox eradication. Thus, the most difficult and problematical areas and years are still ahead, with programme implementation notably hampered by its reliance on a heat-labile vaccine whose efficacy leaves much to be desired and clumsy diagnostic tools. Fortunately, however, research has begun to appear on the programme's agenda. While we all hope that the programme will be successful, there is much yet to be learned and to be applied before success can be assured.

However, an international commitment has been made and high priority must be given to meeting these goals. A failure, especially in achieving poliomyelitis eradication, could as certainly call into question the credibility of the public health profession as did the collapse of the disastrous malaria eradication effort.

As we contemplate the future, is it necessary or even desirable to restrict ourselves to the narrow question of what disease should next be eradicated or eliminated? Through implementation of the smallpox, poliomyelitis and guinea-worm programmes, innovative breakthroughs have been made in organizing large-scale nationwide campaigns; in devising new methods for approaching and mobilizing communities; in developing effective national surveillance networks and in using the data in evolving better strategies; in fostering effective and relevant research programmes to facilitate disease control; and in mobilizing support at international, national and local levels.

I see these approaches as key steps in revolutionizing and revitalizing public health. Implicit in these new approaches is the setting of measurable goals and a willingness to look at all alternative methods for achieving them without assuming, as we so often have, that every intervention, every vaccine, every drug must somehow be directed or dispensed by some sort of primary health centre. These new initiatives and new approaches are of special relevance as we endeavour to deal with tuberculosis, leprosy, and micronutrient deficiencies such as iodine and Vitamin A. Likewise, use of albendazole, ivermectin and praziquantel on a strategically targeted community-wide basis could have a profound effect on many types of symptomatic parasitic disease (20). None of these are conditions to be eradicated in our lifetimes but they are diseases in which far more substantial progress could be made than we are now making while relying primarily on one-on-one traditional curative treatment. As time progresses, it may become apparent that certain of these diseases might warrant an eradication effort or might warrant one if better tools could be made available.

In looking to the future, however, I believe it is critical that we should not be blinded to a range of new public health programme paradigms by staring too fixedly at the blinding beacon of a few eradication dreams.

References

1. **Fenner F et al.** *Smallpox and its eradication.* Geneva, World Health Organization, 1988.
2. Can infectious diseases be eradicated? Symposium papers. *Reviews of infectious diseases*, 1982, **4**: 913–984.
3. **Fenner F.** Global eradication of smallpox. *Reviews of infectious diseases*, 1982, **4**: 916–922.
4. **Henderson DA.** A successful eradication campaign: discussion. *Reviews of infectious diseases*, 1982, **4**: 923–924.
5. **World Health Organization.** Archival records. Tables, by country and year, were developed during the smallpox programme, which indicate the levels of support and donors. At the end of the programme, all the files were given over to WHO Archives.
6. **Henderson DA.** Primary health care as a practical means for measles control. *Reviews of infectious diseases*, 1983, **5**: 606–607.
7. **Goethe T et al.** Methods for the surveillance of endemic treponematoses and sero-epidemiological investigations of "disappearing diseases". *Bulletin of the World Health Organization,* 1972, **46**: 1–14.
8. **Hinman AR, Hopkins DR.** Lessons from previous eradication programs. In: Dowdle WR, Hopkins DR. eds. *The eradication of infectious diseases: report of the Dahlen Workshop on the Eradication of Infectious Diseases.* Clichester, John Wiley & Sons, 1988: 19–32.
9. **Yekutiel P.** Lessons from the big eradication campaigns. *World health forum*, 1981, **2**: 465–490.
10. *Malaria control in developing countries. Where does it stand? What is the U.S. role?* Washington, D.C., U.S. General Accounting Office, 1982 (Document ID 82-27).
11. **Jeffrey GM.** Malaria control in the twentieth century. *American journal of tropical medicine and hygiene*, 1976, **25**: 361–371.
12. **Farid MA.** The malaria program — from euphoria to anarchy. *World health forum*, 1981, **1**: 8–33.
13. **Pampana EJ.** *A textbook of malaria eradication.* London, Oxford University Press, 1963.
14. **Hecker AC et al.** Field work with a stable freeze-dried vaccine prepared in monolayers of primary rabbit kidney cells. *Symposia Series in Immunobiological Standardization*, Vol. 19. Basel, Karger, 1973: 187–195.
15. **Hecker AC et al.** Large-scale use of freeze-dried smallpox vaccine prepared in primary cultures of rabbit kidney cells. *Bulletin of the World Health Organization*, 1976, **54**: 279–284.
16. **Hopkins DR et al.** Dracunculiasis eradication: almost a reality. *American journal of tropical medicine and hygiene*, 1997, **57**: 252–259.
17. **de Quadros C et al.** Polio eradication from the western hemisphere. *Annual reviews of public health*, 1992, **13**: 239–252.
18. **Henderson DA et al.** Design for immunization programs in the developing countries. *International Conference of the Application of Vaccines against Viral, Rickettsial and Bacterial Diseases of Man*, Washington, DC, Pan American Health Organization, 1971: 623–635.
19. **Henderson DA.** The miracle of vaccination. *Notes and records of the Royal Society of London*, 1997, **5**: 235–245.
20. **Warren KS.** An integrated system for the control of the major human helminth parasites. *Acta Leidensia*, 1990, **1/2**: 433–442.

The principles of disease elimination and eradication

Walter R. Dowdle[1]

The Dahlem Workshop discussed the hierarchy of possible public health interventions in dealing with infectious diseases, which were defined as control, elimination of disease, elimination of infections, eradication, and extinction. The indicators of eradicability were the availability of effective interventions and practical diagnostic tools and the essential need for humans in the life-cycle of the agent. Since health resources are limited, decisions have to be made as to whether their use for an elimination or eradication programme is preferable to their use elsewhere. The costs and benefits of global eradication programmes concern direct effects on morbidity and mortality and consequent effects on the health care system. The success of any disease eradication initiative depends strongly on the level of societal and political commitment, with a key role for the World Health Assembly. Eradication and ongoing programmes constitute potentially complementary approaches to public health. Elimination and eradication are the ultimate goals of public health, evolving naturally from disease control. The basic question is whether these goals are to be achieved in the present or some future generation.

Introduction

Elimination and eradication of human disease have been the subject of numerous conferences, symposia, workshops, planning sessions, and public health initiatives for more than a century. Although the malaria, yellow fever, and yaws eradication programmes of earlier years were unsuccessful, they contributed greatly to a better understanding of the biological, social, political, and economic complexities of achieving the ultimate goal in disease control. Smallpox has now been eradicated and programmes are currently under way to eradicate poliomyelitis and guinea-worm disease.

In 1993, the International Task Force for Disease Eradication evaluated over 80 potential infectious disease candidates and concluded that six were eradicable (1). In 1997, the World Health Assembly passed a resolution calling for the "elimination of lymphatic filariasis as a public health problem". Also in early 1997, WHO listed leprosy, onchocerciasis, and Chagas disease as being candidates for elimination "as public health problems within ten years".

With this background, the Dahlem Workshop on the Eradication of Infectious Diseases was held in March 1997 (2). The Workshop was unique in that it focused on the science of eradication, with the understanding that the present Atlanta Conference would address specific candidate diseases for elimination or eradication in the context of global health strategies. The Workshop addressed four questions: 1) How is eradication to be defined and what are the biological criteria? 2) What are the criteria for estimating the cost and benefits of disease eradication? 3) What are the societal and political criteria for eradication? and 4) When and how should eradication programmes be implemented?

Definitions

Eradication has been defined in various ways — as extinction of the disease pathogen (3), as elimination of the occurrence of a given disease, even in the absence of all preventive measures (4), as control of an infection to the point at which transmission ceased within a specified area (5), and as reduction of the worldwide incidence of a disease to zero as a result of deliberate efforts, obviating the necessity for further control measures (1). The hierarchy of potential public health efforts in dealing with infectious diseases was discussed at the Dahlem Workshop. Differences in these efforts made a distinction between the disease caused by the infection and the infection itself, the level of reduction achieved for either of these, the requirement for continuation of

[1] Director of Programs, The Task Force for Child Survival and Development, Suite 400, 750 Commerce Drive, Decatur, Georgia 30030, USA.

control efforts, and, finally, the geographical area covered by the intervention efforts and their outcomes. Although definitions outlined below were developed for infectious diseases, those for control and elimination apply to noninfectious diseases as well.

- *Control*: The reduction of disease incidence, prevalence, morbidity or mortality to a locally acceptable level as a result of deliberate efforts; continued intervention measures are required to maintain the reduction. Example: diarrhoeal diseases.

- *Elimination of disease*: Reduction to zero of the incidence of a specified disease in a defined geographical area as a result of deliberate efforts; continued intervention measures are required. Example: neonatal tetanus.

- *Elimination of infections*: Reduction to zero of the incidence of infection caused by a specific agent in a defined geographical area as a result of deliberate efforts; continued measures to prevent reestablishment of transmission are required. Example: measles, poliomyelitis.

- *Eradication*: Permanent reduction to zero of the worldwide incidence of infection caused by a specific agent as a result of deliberate efforts; intervention measures are no longer needed. Example: smallpox.

- *Extinction*: The specific infectious agent no longer exists in nature or in the laboratory. Example: none.

Principal indicators of eradicability

In theory if the right tools were available, all infectious diseases would be eradicable. In reality there are distinct biological features of the organisms and technical factors of dealing with them that make their potential eradicability more or less likely. Today's categorization of a disease as not eradicable can change completely tomorrow, either because research efforts are successful in developing new and effective intervention tools or because those presumed obstructions to eradicability that seemed important in theory prove capable of being overcome in practice. Three indicators were considered to be of primary importance: an effective intervention is available to interrupt transmission of the agent; practical diagnostic tools with sufficient sensitivity and specificity are available to detect levels of infection that can lead to transmission; and humans are essen-

tial for the life-cycle of the agent, which has no other vertebrate reservoir and does not amplify in the environment.

The effectiveness of an intervention tool has both biological and operational dimensions. Elimination validates the effectiveness of an intervention tool, but it does not necessarily make the agent a candidate for eradication. Highly developed levels of sanitation and health systems development may make elimination possible in one geographical area but not in another.

Diagnostic tools also have both biological and operational dimensions. The tools must be sufficiently sensitive and specific to detect infection that can lead to transmission, and also sufficiently simple to be applied globally by laboratories with a wide range of capabilities and resources. Eradication is a much more feasible target of deliberate intervention when humans form an essential component of the agent's life-cycle. An independent reservoir is not an absolute barrier to eradication if it can be targeted with effective intervention tools.

Economic considerations

Meeting the biological criteria is only one step in the decision to embark upon an elimination or eradication programme. Health resources are limited and resources cross sectors. Therefore, decisions have to be made as to whether the use of resources for an elimination or eradication programme is preferable to their use in nonhealth projects, in alternative health interventions, in continued control of the condition, or even in the eradication of other eradicable conditions. All of these decisions necessitate an evaluation of the cost and benefit of eradication and the alternative use of resources. There is no easy answer.

Formal economic analytical techniques are not ideally suited to eradication programmes. It is not clear, for example, how to handle future benefits and cost, particularly long-term effects. Equally unclear is whether and how to discount future effects. Of the available techniques, the Workshop concluded that cost-effectiveness analysis appeared to be most useful when the outcome is expressed in health terms. This technique allows evaluation of disease eradication in comparisons with other health sector projects.

The costs and benefits of global eradication programmes can be grouped into two categories — direct effects and consequent effects. The direct effects of eradication are that no morbidity or mortality due to that disease will ever again occur. Control programmes can cease. The consequent effects are those that impact positively and negatively on the entire health care system. Because of the close interrelationships between eradication programmes and other health programmes, the Workshop concluded that eradication goals and activities should be expressed in the context of overall health services. Explicit efforts should be taken to maximize the effectiveness of both eradication and comprehensive health programmes.

Social and political criteria

A set of social and political criteria was identified by Workshop participants. These and other related factors are summarized as follows:

- The success of a disease eradication initiative, like any public health programme, is largely dependent on the level of societal and political commitment to it from the beginning to the end. Considering the potentially enormous cost of failure, any proposal for eradication should be given intense scrutiny.

- The disease under consideration for eradication must be of recognized public health importance, with broad international appeal, and be perceived as a worthy goal by all levels of society. There must be specific reasons for eradication. The demands for sustained support, high quality performance, and perseverance in an eradication programme increase the risks of failure, with a consequent significant loss of credibility, resources, and health workers' self-confidence.

- A technically feasible intervention and eradication strategy must be identified, field-tested in a defined geographical area, and found effective. The accumulation of success in individual countries or within a region generates the momentum needed for international support.

- Consensus on the priority and justification for the disease must be developed by technical experts, the decision-makers, and the scientific community.

- Political commitment must be gained at the highest levels, following informed discussion at regional and local levels. A clear commitment of resources from international sources is essential from the start. A resolution by the World Health Assembly is a vital booster to the success of any eradication programme.

- An advocacy plan must be prepared and ready for full implementation at global, regional, and national levels. Eradication requires an effective alliance with all potential collaborators and partners. Finally — a recurring theme — the eradication programme must address the issues of equity and be supportive of broader goals that have a positive impact on the health infrastructure to provide a legacy in addition to eradication of the disease.

- Disease eradication programmes are conceptually simple, focusing on one clear and unequivocal outcome. At the same time, however, their implementation is extraordinarily difficult because of the unique global and time-driven operational challenges. The limitations, potential risks, and points of caution for eradication programmes include higher short-term costs, increased risk of failure and the consequences of failure, an inescapable sense of urgency, and diversion of attention and resources from equally or more important health problems that are not eradicable, or even others that may be eradicable. Care must be taken that eradication efforts do not detract or undermine the development of the general health infrastructure. Other limitations are the high vulnerability of eradication programmes to interruption by war and other civil disturbances; the potential that programmes will not address national priorities in all countries, and that some countries will not follow the eradication strategy; the perception of programmes as "donor driven"; placement of excessive, counterproductive pressures and demands upon health workers and others; and the requirement of special attention for countries with inadequate resources and or weak health infrastructure (including hit-and-run strategies).

- The favourable attributes and potential benefits of eradication programmes are a well-defined scope with a clear objective and endpoint, and the duration is limited. Successful eradication programmes produce sustainable improvement in health and provide a high benefit–cost ratio. Eradication programmes are attractive to potential funding sources because they establish high standards of performance for surveillance, logistics, and administrative support; develop well-trained and highly motivated health staff; assist in the development of health services infrastructure including, for example, mobilization of endemic communities; and provide equity in coverage for all affected areas, including urban, rural, and even remote rural areas. They also offer opportunities for other health benefits (e.g. for dracunculiasis eradication: health education and improved water supply), improved coordination among partners and countries, and dialogue across frontiers during war.

- Decisions on initiating a global disease eradication campaign should also take into consideration the ideal sequencing of potentially concurrent campaigns. Eradication programmes consume major human and financial resources. Careful consideration must be given to whether two or more eradication programmes are to be conducted simultaneously or sequentially, or if the target disease is confined to a limited geographical area.

Disease elimination and eradication programmes can be distinguished from ongoing health or disease control programmes by the urgency of the elimination and eradication programmes and the requirement for targeted surveillance, rapid response capability, high standards of performance, and a dedicated focal point at the national level. Eradication and ongoing programmes constitute potentially complementary approaches to public health. There are areas of potential overlap, conflict and synergy that must be recognized and addressed. In many cases the problem is not that eradication activities function too well but that primary health care activities do not function well enough. Efforts are needed to identify and characterize those factors responsible for improved functioning of eradication campaigns, and then apply them to primary health.

Conclusion

In summary, elimination and eradication programmes are laudable goals, but they carry with them an awesome responsibility. There is no room for failure. Careful and deliberate evaluation is a prerequisite before embarking on any programme. Elimination and eradication are the ultimate goals of public health. The only question is whether these goals are to be achieved in the present or some future generation.

References

1. **Centers for Disease Control and Prevention.** Recommendations of the International Task Force for Disease Eradication. *Morbidity and mortality weekly report*, 1993, **42**(RR-16): 1–38.
2. **Dowdle WR, Hopkins DR.** eds. *The eradication of infectious diseases: report of the Dahlem Workshop on the Eradication of Infections Diseases.* Chichester, John Wiley & Sons, 1998.
3. **Cockburn TA.** Eradication of infectious diseases. *Science*, 1996, **133**: 1050–1058.
4. **Soper FL.** Problems to be solved if the eradication of tuberculosis is to be realized. *American journal of public health*, 1962, **52**: 734–745.
5. **Andrews JM, Langmuir AD.** The philosophy of disease eradication. *American journal of public health*, 1963, **53**: 1–6.

Disease eradication and health systems development

B. Melgaard,[1] A. Creese,[2] B. Aylward,[1] J.-M. Olivé,[1] C. Maher,[3] J.-M. Okwo-Bele,[4] & J.W. Lee[1]

This article provides a framework for the design of future eradication programmes so that the greatest benefit accrues to health systems development from the implementation of such programmes. The framework focuses on weak and fragile health systems and assumes that eradication leads to the cessation of the intervention required to eradicate the disease. Five major components of health systems are identified and key elements which are of particular relevance to eradication initiatives are defined. The dearth of documentation which can provide "lessons learned" in this area is illustrated with a brief review of the literature. Opportunities and threats, which can be addressed during the design of eradication programmes, are described and a number of recommendations are outlined. It is emphasized that this framework pertains to eradication programmes but may be useful in attempts to coordinate vertical and horizontal disease control activities for maximum mutual benefits.

Introduction

Strategies for disease control, elimination and eradication are derived primarily from the epidemiological characteristics of the disease, the intervention available, the logistical requirements, and the resource needs. While control measures usually depend on routine services being instituted and maintained in a long-term perspective, eradication activities are characterized as time-limited, often intensive, targeted, and organized in circumscribed programmes with campaign elements as prominent features.

Eradication/elimination programmes (EP) have therefore been considered to be dominated by nonsustainable activities that may bypass or, at worst, even compromise the development of the health sector, especially in the poorer developing countries. Experience from ongoing eradication programmes calls this assessment into question and indicates that they may have positive impacts on health services and systems that stretch beyond the narrow benefits of eradication of a single disease. Taylor & Waldman (1) have stressed that "past polarization between proponents of primary health care and eradication represents an exaggerated example of continuing controversies between vertical and horizontal programs. It is time to admit that this is a false polarization which has become unnecessarily emotional and irrational".

The challenge that arises is to design current and future eradication and elimination programmes in such a way that they provide maximum benefits to national health systems without jeopardizing the eradication efforts. Eradication and elimination activities can make substantial contributions to sustainable health development. This article addresses that challenge.

We describe major elements of health systems, the areas most relevant to eradication and elimination programmes, and identify the key issues that relate to such programmes. Selected major opportunities and threats to health systems are identified in a framework for the design of future eradication initiatives.

The focus is on developing health systems and services in developing countries with weak or fragile health systems, assuming that in countries with strong systems the potential negative effects of eradication efforts are less pronounced.

Health systems and eradication programmes

A national health system can be defined as the set of activities in a country which provide health services to the population and health results. The following

[1] Global Programme on Vaccines and Immunization, World Health Organization, 1211 Geneva 27, Switzerland.

[2] Division of Analysis, Research and Assessment, World Health Organization, 1211 Geneva 27, Switzerland.

[3] Expanded Programme on Immunization, World Health Organization, Regional Office for the Western Pacific, Manila, Philippines.

[4] Expanded Programme on Immunization, World Health Organization, Harare, Zimbabwe

Bulletin of the World Health Organization, 1998, **76** (Suppl. 2): 26–31

are commonly recognized components of health systems (2):

— health policy, regulatory and strategic planning functions;

— definition and development of institutions/organizational arrangements;

— mobilization and allocation of financial resources;

— mobilization and allocation of human resources; and

— management and delivery of health services.

This framework provides a basis for identifying and examining elements of the health systems that pertain to eradication strategies and they offer particular opportunities and/or threats (see Table 1).

Eradication can be defined as "permanent reduction to zero of the worldwide incidence of infection caused by a specific agent as a result of deliberate efforts, intervention measures are no longer needed" (3). The cessation of control measures is important and distinguishes eradication from elimination. It has been argued that this makes eradication particularly favourable in cost–benefit terms. Such savings could be channelled to benefit other areas of health services. The benefits from poliomyelitis eradication in terms of savings on the global health budget has been estimated at US$ 1700 million per year for direct costs only (4). The indirect benefits are considered to be substantially higher.

The sustainability of health systems can be defined as the ability to deliver an appropriate level of benefits for an extended period of time after major financial and technical donor assistance has been terminated. Sustainable health development thus relates to countries where donor assistance is available to the health sector. Since eradication programmes, by definition, aim at being terminated when successful, it follows that the question of sustainability is relevant to health system elements which are not dedicated to eradication initiatives.

Eradication programmes must be implemented even in situations where health systems are weak or absent. The implementation of poliomyelitis eradication in countries afflicted by war has been achieved

Table 1: **Key elements of health systems and examples of the opportunities and threats presented by the implementation of disease eradication or elimination programmes**

Health system element	Examples of the impact of eradication/elimination activities	
	Potential opportunities	Potential threats
Health policy regulatory and strategic planning function	• Policy: strengthening of national health policy development	• Strategic planning: compromising local decision-making
	• Stakeholders: increased transparency and broadened commitment to health	• Imposition of external priorities
Institutional arrangements	• Management systems: systematic introduction of targets and indicators	• Management processes: risk of establishing parallel structures
	• Decentralization: mechanisms for delegating authority to districts	
Financial resources: mobilization and use	• Resource mobilization: improved advocacy and mobilization mechanisms	• Fund-raising and resource allocation: diversion of scarce financial resources
	• Private sector resources: expanded role of private sector in public health	
Human resources: number, mix and quality	• Incentive schemes: introduction of performance-based incentive models	• Human resources: diversion of personnel as opposed to increasing productivity
	• Training: coordination of strong training component with national plans	• Uncoordinated in-service training
Service management and delivery	• Access to services: increased access and utilization of health services	• Service delivery: disruption of routine service delivery
	• Surveillance: establishing surveillance as a key tool in disease control	

by negotiating between warring factions, so that immunization campaigns could be carried out on days of tranquillity. In such situations, eradication activities may contribute to the initiation of new efforts in health system strengthening.

Major issues in health systems development and eradication and elimination programmes

Overall health policy and strategic planning

Central to all national health systems is an overall health policy and the strategic planning required to implement that policy. The policy should reflect the national health priorities based on the proportional burden of disease and available resources, both human and financial, to address those priorities. Ideally, the strategic planning to reach those goals includes the delineation of specific objectives with detailed strategies, the implementation of which can be monitored through both health outcomes and process indicators. Unfortunately, in many countries, particularly those in the most difficult circumstances, health policies are often vague or outdated, if they exist at all. These same countries are frequently the last reservoirs of organisms targeted for eradication. Since donor agencies may exert a substantial influence on the policy development in such countries, stakeholders in eradication initiatives can temporarily exert a strong effect on this process.

Eradication/elimination programmes are characterized by clearly defined policies and strategies. As a result, the adoption and implementation of an eradication programme can facilitate the need for a country to establish defined health goals with specific strategies and indicators for evaluation and monitoring. Basic eradication policies are often generated from the experience of countries and regions with good health systems. These policies are then adopted by the global community when the feasibility of the EP target has been demonstrated. Subsequent adoption in poor countries can be influenced by the strong promotion of the global policy as its implementation is a prerequisite for the successful achievement of targets.

Eradication strategies are generally standardized with limited leeway for national adaptation and interpretation. Despite endorsing the goal of poliomyelitis eradication, some countries are reluctant to implement the WHO-recommended strategies, especially countries in Africa. For example, Ghana initially resisted vertical disease control initiatives including eradication because they were considered detrimental to overall health systems development (5). Opportunities to strengthen the national health policy process may be missed when eradication strategies are advocated for their own sake.

Organization of health systems: structures and processes

National health systems require an established structure with well-defined lines of authority, responsibility and accountability. Eradication programmes give an emphasis to the need for strong management capacity and processes. Countries with a good health management structure can exploit the eradication initiative to further strengthen that structure. In countries where this structure is fragile or particularly weak, an EP could undermine pre-existing lines of management authority if a separate system is established in parallel. The management demands of an EP may divert staff time away from routine programmes, as in Mozambique where a large share of the EPI management time was used to plan NIDs. However, a negative effect is by no means universal. In Cambodia, the planning and implementation of the first NIDs in the early 1990s provided a mechanism by which a recently revitalized Ministry of Health could demonstrate its capacity to conduct nationwide health initiatives while strengthening the weak lines of responsibility.

Historically, EPs required the creation of new health management structures in many countries, because of the lack of an existing capacity. More recent initiatives have been implemented within the existing health management set-up even though it may be less developed. This may contribute to overall strengthening of the management capacity beyond the programme. The management of EPs is centrally driven and often leaves limited scope for change and adaptation by district authorities. Innovation at the peripheral level to successfully achieve nationally established performance indicators remains possible. These efforts can, and do, exploit the commitment and energy that develops among health staff and in the community for other health activities. To capitalize on the opportunities for health systems development the eradication strategies must concentrate on existing organizational arrangements, assess their strengths and weaknesses, and ensure that the management of the EP is designed to strengthen established structures.

Financial resources: mobilization and use

Health systems require substantial resources, the majority of which must be identified locally, for

Fig. 1. **Per capita costs of selected health interventions compared with average public expenditure on health in low-income countries.**

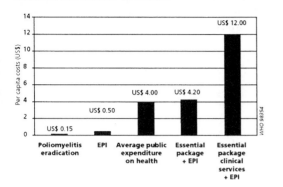

both capital and recurrent costs. Eradication programmes utilize relatively less funds (in comparison to overall health systems development), primarily from external sources in the poorest countries, and for a time-limited period. The relationship is illustrated in Fig. 1 for poliomyelitis.

There is a widespread perception that the funds used for eradication programmes divert resources that would be available for health systems development in a country. There is a paucity of hard data with which to evaluate this point, but both recent and previous eradication initiatives have been capable of raising substantial additional resources compared with the underfunded routine health services. Although the capacity to raise substantial resources for eradication is partly due to the inherent nature of such initiatives, these programmes may provide lessons in resource mobilization for the health sector, since they are more efficient in both the raising and use of resources.

Gyldmark & Alban (6) emphasize the need for economic evaluations of eradication programmes, with particular attention paid to the potential opportunity costs of using resources on eradication than on other more urgent health care problems. However, a sizable proportion of the resources that go to EPs might not be available for development aid at all, much less for the health sector. Striking examples of this are Rotary International's US$ 450 million for poliomyelitis eradication and SmithKline Beecham's recent donation of drug supplies worth more than US$ 2000 million for lymphatic filariasis eradication.

The actual public spending from national sources on eradication activities in poor countries is small; in the poorest countries it is estimated that the maximum public sector spending on poliomyelitis eradication in a year will be US$ 0.025 to US$ 0.05

per capita. It can be argued that the cost for the poorest countries should be covered by the donor community, especially since they will benefit from successful eradication (7).

Private sector involvement and volunteer contributions in-kind are much more common in eradication programmes and remain an undertapped source for the health sector. These programmes may be a model to both central and peripheral level health authorities for promoting public–private sector cooperation to achieve health goals.

Human resources: number, mix and quality

Even in those countries where human resource planning provides for the proper number and mix of personnel, the effectiveness is often compromised by the low performance common to the underfunded public sector. This affects the productivity of the health labour force. The impact of introducing an eradication programme, with its substantial human resource requirements, into such a setting must be considered.

Increased staff resources (in time if not in actual personnel) are required at both the central and peripheral levels for eradication activities. Whether these extra resources are met by expanding staff at the central level or increasing the work load for all existing staff, there remains a concern that this could in turn divert staff time from routine tasks. Unfortunately, there is only anecdotal information on this issue. There are no data to determine whether the introduction and implementation of an eradication programme increases the productivity of the health sector as opposed to diverting energies to the detriment of other programmes. Evaluating the opportunity costs of any new programme in a developing country setting is complicated by the generally low productivity of the public sector.

The Taylor Commission (8) highlighted both the commitment and positive attitude of staff during poliomyelitis eradication in the Americas but also the frustration over the prioritization of staff time to this disease. The incentives which are sometimes introduced for certain eradication functions, such as surveillance, seldom if ever exist in the routine services. Such rewards have attracted staff to eradication and increased their commitment, while discouraging staff who are not involved. In the more recent programmes, however, rewards are usually foregone in preference to reimbursement of actual costs — possibly a feasible model for improving the productivity of the health sector in general.

Training for eradication is very target oriented and generally dedicated, but often carried out with little attention to other health training activities.

These, similarly, tend to be uncoordinated, thereby compromising the delivery of routine services.

Service management and delivery

The equity problem of ensuring access to services for all population groups is particularly acute in countries where curative services in major population centres receive priority. Countries with fragile civil institutions and with limited financial resources are especially susceptible. Eradication strategies must be designed to increase access to and utilization of services beyond that normally achieved by routine services.

To achieve this goal, eradication efforts often include campaign elements. While the interventions are usually specific to the eradication initiative, the campaigns may offer opportunities for the addition of other interventions. Although such strategies can deliver health interventions to the entire population, the impact on other health priorities must be considered. Routine coverage has been reported to drop immediately following national immunization days in some countries, but subsequently has usually climbed back to similar if not higher levels.

Routine information systems are often fragmented and unreliable and improvements can be compromised by the development and consolidation of surveillance for eradication, if it is initiated as a parallel and specific activity. This was a concern when of the surveillance system for poliomyelitis eradication was established in Cambodia (9), but the system was gradually expanded to include other diseases. Similarly the poliomyelitis surveillance system played an important role in the cholera epidemic in Latin America in the late 1980s. The surveillance approach to disease control has significant potential for integration and expansion to other priority diseases, as exemplified by the integrated disease surveillance system being promoted in the African region with poliomyelitis surveillance as one of a number of central functions.

Performance monitoring is rare in the health sector but common in eradication programmes. A broader adaptation of performance indicators may enhance the quality of other health services.

Conclusions and recommendations

Eradication and elimination programmes offer both opportunities and threats to health systems development. While early eradication efforts were imple-mented as vertical operations — often in the absence of a service delivery system — more recent programmes have increasingly utilized and worked within the frame of the existing health system (10, 11). This has sometimes led to diversion of resources and disputes over the priority accorded to eradication when a global objective is pursued in countries which do not share this prioritization.

Increasingly, evidence is being collected on the beneficial impacts of eradication efforts on the health sector and it has become apparent that carefully designed programmes may produce benefits beyond the eradication goal (8, 12). The framework presented in this article provides guidance for the design of future programmes to maximize the support to national health systems development and thus increase the impact on the health status of the populations.

The framework is applicable primarily to eradication initiatives but may be adapted to other targeted ("vertical") health programmes in order to strengthen the coordination of health systems development and disease control efforts for mutual benefit. The following main recommendations are put forward:

- EP policy and strategy development should be used to stimulate and support national health policies development and become components of these.

- Stakeholders in eradication should use their influence to promote health systems development as a secondary objective of eradication.

- Management systems for eradication should be designed with reference to existing systems and gradually integrated into these.

- Strengthening of existing organizational structures and management processes, including wide use of performance indicators, should receive priority over the establishment of new systems.

- Donor commitment to eradication should be extended to other health system investments.

- Savings from cessation of eradication programme activities should accrue to health sector development following achievement of eradication.

- Specific training activities should be planned and coordinated with other training programmes.

- Strategies for service delivery for eradication should be more widely used by other health services.

- Surveillance should be expanded as the most essential function of disease control.

References

1. **Taylor CE, Waldman RJ.** Designing eradication programs to strengthen primary health care. In: Dowdle WR, Hopkins DR. eds. *The eradication of infectious disease: report of the Dahlem Workshop on the Eradication of Infectious Diseases.* Chichester, John Wiley & Sons, 1998: 145–155.
2. World Health Organization. *Challenges and strategies for health systems development.* Unpublished WHO document HDP/97.3, 1997.
3. **Centers for Disease Control and Prevention.** Recommendations of the International Task Force for Disease Eradication. *Morbidity and mortality weekly report,* 1993, **43**: 1–38.
4. **Bart KJ, Foulds J, Partriarca P.** Global eradication of poliomyelitis: benefit-cost analysis. *Bulletin of the World Health Organization,* 1996, **74**: 35–45.
5. **Kwadwo-Amofah G.** The coordination of vertical programmes and the development of integrated health systems in Ghana: a regional perspective. In: *National Meeting on the Coordination and Integration of Health Programmes and Services in Ghana, 14–16 January 1991, Ministry of Health Accra.* Unpublished WHO document, WHO/SHS/DHS91.2, 1991.
6. **Gyldmark M, Alban A.** An economic perspective on programs proposed for eradication of infectious diseases. In: Dowdle WR, Hopkins DR. eds. *The eradication of infectious diseases: report of the Dahlem Workshop on the Eradication of Infectious Diseases.* Chichester, John Wiley & Sons, 1998: 91–106.
7. **Taylor CE, Cutts F, Taylor ME.** Ethical dilemmas in current planning for polio eradication. *American journal of public health,* 1997, **87**: 922–925.
8. **Taylor Commission.** The impact of the Expanded Program on Immunization and the Polio Eradication Initiative on health systems in the Americas. Washington, DC, Pan American Health Organization, 1995.
9. **Nareth L et al.** Establishing acute flaccid paralysis surveillance under difficult circumstances: lessons learned in Cambodia. *Journal of infectious diseases,* 1997, **175** (Suppl.1): 173–175.
10. **Fenner F et al.** *Smallpox and its eradication.* Geneva, World Health Organization, 1988.
11. **Yekutiel P.** Lessons from the big eradication campaigns. *World health forum,* 1981, **2**: 465–481.
12. **Aylward RB et al.** Disease eradication initiatives and general health services: ensuring common principles lead to mutual benefits. In: Dowdle WR, Hopkins RD. eds. *The eradication of infectious diseases: report of the Dahlem Workshop on the Eradication of Infectious Diseases.* Chichester, John Wiley & Sons, 1998: 61–74.

PERSPECTIVES FROM ONGOING PROGRAMMES

Perspectives from micronutrient malnutrition elimination/eradication programmes

B.A. Underwood[1]

Micronutrient malnutrition cannot be eradicated, but the elimination and control of iron, vitamin A and iodine deficiencies and their health-related consequences as public health problems are currently the targets of global programmes. Remarkable progress is occurring in the control of goitre and xerophthalmia, but iron-deficiency anaemia (IDA) has been less responsive to prevention and control efforts. Subclinical consequences of micronutrient deficiencies, i.e. "hidden hunger", include compromised immune functions that increase the risk of morbidity and mortality, impaired cognitive development and growth, and reduced reproductive and work capacity and performance. The implications are obvious for human health and national and global economic and social development. Mixes of affordable interventions are available which, when appropriately adapted to resource availability and context, are proven to be effective. These include both food-based interventions, particularly fortification programmes, such as salt iodization, and use of concentrated micronutrient supplements. A mix of accompanying programmes for infection control, community participation, including education, communication and information exchange, and private sector involvement are lessons learned for overcoming deterrents and sustaining progress towards elimination.

Background

Micronutrients are essential vitamins and minerals that are needed in small amounts for various physiological functions, but which cannot be made in sufficient quantities in the body. Although several nutrients meet this definition, only three — iron, vitamin A and iodine — are currently major targets for public health programmes to control the deficiency and prevent any health-related consequences. Other micronutrient deficiencies, e.g. zinc, folate, and possibly vitamin B_{12}, could become of public health concern as more is learned about their prevalence and health consequences. Because the body cannot be stimulated to produce essential micronutrients or be made less dependent on them, they must be provided regularly in the food or through supplements. The need for some micronutrients, however, can be lessened by correcting any factors that decrease efficient absorption, utilization and conservation, e.g. by menu adjustments to improve bioavailability and control of infectious disease.

From a global perspective, micronutrient malnutrition cannot be eradicated and is unlikely to be eliminated, as defined by zero incidences, even if control measures are continued. But the problem can be reduced to an acceptable public health level by deliberate efforts, which will need to continue for the foreseeable future. Using this definition of elimination, i.e. elimination as a problem of public health significance, iodine-deficiency disease (IDD) is on the horizon for elimination, followed by vitamin A deficiency (VAD) and iron deficiency (ID). A range of possible interventions exist for the elimination of these three deficiencies, some of which could be linked to other public health efforts, e.g. immunization programmes that include distribution of supplements to vulnerable groups, parasite elimination programmes aiming to improve efficiency of iron metabolism, and diarrhoea control programmes that enhance vitamin A conservation. Depending on the mix of control strategies, the effort applied to each, and the prevailing social and economic levels of development, the elimination of other micronutrient deficiencies could also be addressed.

Magnitude of micronutrient malnutrition

It is fallacious to estimate the magnitude of a health problem due to micronutrient malnutrition using extant signs of deficiency. This approach was characteristic of pre-1990 thinking and did not excite political concern or broad-based interventions. While relatively few persons are clinically affected, subclinical deficits — "hidden hunger" — are more pervasive, and include consequences that potentially compromise immune functions (morbidity and

---

[1] Food and Nutrition Board, Institute of Medicine, National Academy of Sciences, Washington, DC 20418, USA.

mortality, cognitive development (school performance and mental achievement) and growth, reproductive and work capacity, and performances (achieving potentials and productivity). The consequences of micronutrient malnutrition therefore extend beyond individuals and families to whole communities and nations. The magnitude of the problem is reasonably firm when estimates are based on clinical signs but less firm when based on those whose health is compromised by subclinical effects. Early in the 1990s, WHO estimated that deficiencies of iron, iodine, and vitamin A influenced the health of 2000 million, 1500 million, and 250 million persons, respectively; often these deficiencies overlapped in the population groups affected (1).

Causes and consequences

Signs of micronutrient deficiencies have been noted in ancient art and literature, and efforts to treat and control the problems are recorded in medical lore that long preceded an understanding of their basis (2). Through the ages, but particularly during the twentieth century and especially the last quarter of this century, scientific discoveries have elucidated the causes and broad-ranging consequences of deficiencies of iron, vitamin A, and iodine. Epidemiological studies have identified vulnerable groups and factors associated with prevalence, and have provided reasonable global prevalence estimates. National and community intervention trials have demonstrated effective, affordable, population-based solutions. None the less, micronutrient malnutrition has not been eliminated as a global problem. The most notable barriers to elimination are not the lack of scientific understanding but operational deterrents, including absence of political resolve at all levels (not just at the top), ineffective use of financial and human resources, and lack of intervention strategies packaged in a mix of validated effective programmes with appropriate effort given to each intervention. The deterrents can be overcome by deliberate global and local efforts. This conference is an important global effort to generate resolve, resources, and a framework for developing, implementing and monitoring appropriate strategies for universal sustained disease elimination. However, it is unlikely that a "one-size-fits-all" global solution will be found at national and local levels. The exception may be iodine-deficiency disorders, which are showing a remarkable response to universal salt iodization (USI). For vitamin A and iron deficiencies, however, successful elimination will be sustainable only when people are able to procure and are willing to consume diets, including fortified foods, that contain micronutrients in adequate quantity and quality, or to procure supplements during periods of increased physiological need or other difficult nutrition situations.

Progress towards control

Global programme initiatives taken in the last decade are making an impact. Recent monitoring shows progress in control of clinical and subclinical forms of micronutrient malnutrition, particularly of iodine and vitamin A deficiencies (2, 3). Goitre and xerophthalmia rates — markers of clinical deficiency — are declining, and shifts in urinary iodine concentrations and serum retinol distribution levels — markers of subclinical deficiencies — are shifting towards adequate levels, especially for iodine. Unfortunately, there is less evidence of global progress in controlling iron deficiency and iron deficiency anaemia (IDA). However, the true magnitude of global progress during the 1990s has been inadequately evaluated because there are a limited number of post-intervention, repeat biological assessment surveys, particularly for vitamin A and iron (4). For iodine, post-intervention surveys, especially in Latin America, show that IDD has been eliminated in several countries, e.g. Bolivia, Ecuador and Peru, and that the global prevalence has been reduced from about 30% early in the decade to 14% in 1997.

Corroboration of progress comes from process indicators (usually easier to monitor than biological indicators), which show growing programme-coverage achievements for both iodine and vitamin A (4). Control programmes for IDD in developing countries began with the use of iodine concentrate (initially by injection, and later orally), through one-to-one delivery programmes with slow and costly progress. More recently, accelerated and cost-effective progress has been achieved through USI in places where this programme has been mandated, monitored, and enforced, even at the level of community managed enterprises in hard-to-reach areas. Iodized salt is now reaching remote areas in developing countries, where only in isolated situations and emergencies is there a need for injection or oral delivery of concentrates. Sustained control, however, depends on institutionalizing salt iodization, product quality assurance, and continued effective surveillance.

Progress towards control of xerophthalmia is not easily attributed to a single intervention approach. Periodic universal or targeted distribution of high-dose supplements is the single most used intervention approach and coverage has increased and undoubtedly contributed towards control. Although the cost of the supplement is small (US$ 0.02–0.03), the human resource cost to achieve and sustain high coverage on a repetitive basis is considerable and competes with other health service needs. The recent linking of vitamin A distribution to national immunization days (NIDs) focused on poliomyelitis eradication or to measles immunieation, supplemented by a mid-year campaign (micronutrient days), has achieved high coverage (4). However, the sustainability of a campaign approach is in question because special immunization days are expected to be phased out, and because campaigns to support single health issues that must be repeated biannually are costly in money and manpower. Even in Indonesia, where vitamin A supplements have dominated national control efforts since 1974 and xerophthalmia, i.e. clinical deficiency, was declared to be under control in 1994, low serum retinol levels have persisted among over 50% of preschool-aged children. Thus, to rid a country of all the consequences of VAD, i.e. to eliminate it as a public health problem, requires a more diversified strategy, including control of infectious disease and improvement of the diet (5).

There is little evidence of global progress in controlling ID — or even IDA — in developing countries where prevalence rates are high. Lack of compliance with daily supplementation regimens, and inhibitors to bioavailability from local foods and fortified products have been major, but potentially surmountable, constraints. In some countries, such as Venezuela, iron fortification of wheat and corn flour has effectively halted a trend towards increased prevalence of deficiency due to inadequate food consumption as a result of a declining economy (6). However, the general level of bioavailability of iron from Venezuelan diets is considerably greater than that in, for example, South Asia, where fortification alone is unlikely to control the problem. Indeed, the wide range in the bioavailability of non-haem iron from diets typical of different cultures where anaemia is prevalent again argues for broad-based interventions, which in many situations would require attacking the contributing causes such as hookworm, schistosomiasis and malaria infections.

Lessons from ongoing programmes

The major factors noted above for progress, or lack thereof, in elimination of micronutrient malnutrition argue for holistic strategies. Such strategies usually require a mix of direct and indirect interventions based on modifications in the quantity and quality of diets, including use of fortified food products, supplementation, and public health measures, as well as education and awareness campaigns (5). On the surface the case for control of IDD would appear to be an exception, i.e. a single mandated fortification programme applied in underdeveloped countries appears to have worked. And, based on experience in industrialized countries, such as the USA, Switzerland, and Austria, where salt iodization has controlled IDD for over half a century, the success will be sustainable as long as the control measure continues. The tenuous political and economic circumstances existing in many developing countries, however, and current experience in some of them, confirm that legislation alone may be inadequate unless coupled with demand creation and change in human behaviour. Information, education, and communication (IEC) are important at political and consumer levels to sustain support for enforcement, quality control, and surveillance.

Are there other lessons from the remarkable success in moving towards IDD elimination that are applicable to other micronutrients? To consider this question, it is prudent to compare briefly the epidemiology of the micronutrient deficiencies as relevant to selection of intervention measures. In addition to fortified food products, increasing the quantity or variety of food grown locally in endemically deficient areas can contribute to elimination of both vitamin A and iron deficiencies, but not iodine. Controlling infectious diseases will have a minor influence on the prevalence of IDD or its severity because ingested iodine is readily absorbed and assimilated even in the presence of illness, and virtually irrespective of other food items. In contrast, disease control and food selection and preparation will significantly influence absorption and utilization of both vitamin A and iron. For all three micronutrients, past failures have led to an awareness of the importance of IEC strategies to accompany all interventions, even those of mandated fortification. Where consumers have a choice they must be convinced that the fortified products bring benefits to them, and where they do not have a choice, i.e. mandated universal fortification, politicians must continually be reminded of the benefits — political, economic and health — of effective programmes and their continuation even when national financial difficulties occur. A very recent example comes from the mandated, universal vitamin A sugar fortification legislation in Guatemala, which was temporarily rescinded in early January 1998 for political rather than health reasons. Previously, sugar fortification had also been stopped for economic reasons and it took several years to reinstate the programme. Fortunately the recent stoppage was temporary because a public and international outcry resulted in a quick reversal of the decision that came forth from an informed group of advocates and consumers. Hence, I argue that IEC is a crucial part of strategies for sustainability.

Because the etiology of vitamin A and iron deficiencies are more complex than for iodine, it is less realistic on a global basis to hope for similar success from fortification alone for the control of vitamin A and iron malnutrition, or to rely only on repetitive distribution of high-dose nutrient supplements. Both approaches are likely to be needed in the elimination battle. Solutions based on food production and dietary diversification and modification, which also have proven effective in some circumstances, have received least support as interventions partly because they are difficult to monitor and evaluate, require more resource inputs, take longer to implement, and are slower to demonstrate improvement in micronutrient status. None the less, recent studies demonstrate feasible means to speed the process of dietary diversification through well-designed intensive social marketing and education techniques that include building support structures to reinforce behavioural changes. The studies showed improved micronutrient status sustained after the intensive intervention had terminated. A key element to success has been community participation.

This analysis would suggest that the lessons from IDD control that are transferable to other micronutrients apply primarily to fortification process issues, including forming lasting government–private sector partnerships which respect the need for incentives and corporate benefit, in addition to creating a sense of social responsibility involving IEC. In contrast, more limited information from food-based programmes indicated that people participation and ownership are key elements if changed behaviours are desired outcomes.

I challenge programme planners and implementers to analyse the problem of elimination of micronutrient malnutrition based on the broadly accepted premises and global facts shown below.

- The causes and consequences, risk factors and context determinants and prevalence are sufficiently known to warrant public health actions.

- A "tool kit" of proven efficacious interventions exists, most of which individually have been shown to be affordable and effective under controlled community trial conditions, and to a limited degree in community settings.

- The remarkable progress in IDD control has occurred because a single cost-effective tool well matched to the global problem has received broad political, financial and technical support, i.e. USI,

and it is expected that sustainable elimination as a public health problem will occur probably in the next decade. We need to evaluate critical elements leading to success in this programme and extract those that might be applicable to other micronutrient control strategies.

- Despite progress in controlling vitamin A and iron deficiencies, the goal of elimination is more distant because a less simplistic global solution is in hand. The most effective mix of solutions depends not only on availability but also the social, economic and ecological settings in which they will be implemented, and the prospects for sustainability in the short and long term. Context-specific, flexible strategies are needed to adjust the mix of solutions and level of effort given to each as overall development evolves and situations move towards elimination.

Conclusions

Control of some micronutrient deficiencies has been a by-product of economic, social, and ecological development, or the equitable distribution of social and economic resources, but these development processes are often slow to evolve in the developing world. It is unacceptable, however, to allow the consequences of micronutrient malnutrition to continue where development is slow because affordable solutions are available. Therefore, although elimination of micronutrient malnutrition should be seen as a development issue, it can be facilitated through deliberate intervention efforts, including — but not limited to — the use of vitamin and mineral supplements. The challenge is to select the correct mix for every situation.

References

1. **World Health Organization.** *National strategies for overcoming micronutrient malnutrition.* Geneva, 1992 (unpublished document A45/17).
2. **Underwood BA.** Micronutrient malnutrition: Is it being eliminated? *Nutrition today,* 1998, **33**: 121–129.
3. **Administrative Committee on Coordination/Subcommittee on Nutrition (ACC/SCN).** *Third world nutrition report,* 1997.
4. **UNICEF.** *State of the world's children 1998.* New York. UNICEF, 1998
5. **Committee on Micronutrient Deficiencies, Board on International Health & Food and Nutrition Board, Institute of Medicine.** *Prevention of micronutrient deficiencies. Tools for policymakers and public health workers* (Howson CP et al. eds.). Washington, DC, National Academy Press, 1998.
6. **Laryisse et al.** Early response to the impact of iron fortification in the Venezuelan population. *American journal of clinical nutrition,* 1996, **64**: 903–907.

Perspectives from the dracunculiasis eradication programme*

D.R. Hopkins[1]

After a slow beginning in association with the International Drinking Water Supply and Sanitation Decade (1981–1990), the global Dracunculiasis Eradication Programme has reduced the incidence of dracunculiasis by nearly 97%, from an estimated 3.2 million cases in 1986 to less than 100000 cases in 1997. Over half of the remaining cases are in Sudan. In addition, the programme has already produced many indirect benefits such as improved agricultural production and school attendance, extensive provision of clean drinking-water, mobilization of endemic communities, and improved care of infants. Most workers in the campaign have other responsibilities in their communities or ministries of health besides dracunculiasis eradication.

Introduction

Dracunculiasis (guinea-worm disease) is an infection in humans caused by the parasite *Dracunculus medinensis*, which is contracted by drinking contaminated water from ponds, step wells or other open stagnant sources. After about 1 year, the 0.6–0.9-m long adult female worm emerges slowly through the victim's skin in an attempt to deposit immature larvae in water. Some of the larvae are eaten by a tiny crustacean or copepod (*Cyclops*), in which the larvae undergo two moults within about 2–3 weeks. People are infected when they drink water containing the copepods with infective larvae. Each infection lasts 1 year, and there is no protective immunity. Humans are the only definitive hosts of *D. medinensis*, and they are infected only by drinking contaminated water.

Once a person is infected, there is no treatment to kill the parasite before it emerges a year later. The disease can be prevented, however, by teaching people to filter their drinking-water through a finely woven cloth or to boil their water if they can afford it; by educating communities to keep people with emerging worms from entering sources of drinking-water; by applying the cyclopsicide temephos to contaminated sources every 4 weeks; or by providing safe sources of drinking-water from borehole wells (*1*).

Dracunculiasis is rarely fatal, but the pain and secondary infections associated with the emerging worm incapacitate infected persons for periods averaging 8 weeks. The worms emerge on the lower leg and are the sole evidence of the infection; however, they may emerge from any part of the body, and a dozen or more may emerge simultaneously from some infected persons. Over half of a village's population may be infected at the same time, and the outbreaks usually coincide with the planting or harvest season and the school year. Thus the impact of this quintessentially rural disease manifests itself in mass temporary crippling, which in turn substantially reduces agricultural production and greatly increases school absenteeism (*2*). Other indirect adverse effects have been documented on infant nutrition, child care and childhood immunizations (*3, 4*).

The eradication campaign

The global campaign to eradicate dracunculiasis began with an initiative at the Centers for Disease Control and Prevention (CDC) in 1980, which took advantage of the impending International Drinking Water Supply and Sanitation Decade (1981–1990) (*5*). It was not known how many people were infected by dracunculiasis at that time, but a WHO estimate put the number at about 10 million (*6*). In addition to India and Pakistan, 16 countries in sub-Saharan Africa were known to be infected (Benin, Burkina Faso, Cameroon, Chad, Côte d'Ivoire, Ethiopia, Ghana, Kenya, Mali, Mauritania, Niger, Nigeria, Senegal, Sudan, Togo, and Uganda). Yemen was discovered to be endemic in 1994. In 1986, Watts published a country-by-country estimate of the numbers of persons infected, which totalled 3.2 million (*7*). Over 120 million persons were judged to be at risk of the infection in Africa alone.

Despite the adoption of dracunculiasis eradication in 1981 as a sub-goal of the Water and Sanitation Decade, one of the main goals of which was to pro-

* The views expressed in this article are those of the author and may differ from those held by WHO.

[1] Associate Executive Director, The Carter Center, Atlanta, GA, USA.

vide safe drinking-water to all who did not yet have it, support for the eradication programme was exceedingly slow in coming. In 1982 the US National Research Council, CDC, and the US Agency for International Development convened an international Workshop on Opportunities for Control of Dracunculiasis in Washington in collaboration with WHO. In 1986, the World Health Assembly adopted its first resolution calling for the "elimination" of dracunculiasis; the first African Regional Conference on Dracunculiasis Eradication met in Niamey, Niger; and The Carter Center (Global 2000) and CDC began assisting the eradication programme in Pakistan. African ministers of health resolved at Brazzaville in 1988 to eradicate dracunculiasis by the end of 1995, a target date which was endorsed by the World Health Assembly in 1991. An international donors' conference co-sponsored by The Carter Center, UNDP and UNICEF at Lagos in 1989 mobilized US$ 10 million for the global programme. As illustrated elsewhere (8), however, by the end of the Water Decade, only four of the 18 endemic countries (India, Pakistan, Ghana, and Nigeria) had begun implementing national eradication programmes, and 10 of the countries only began implementing their programmes in 1993 or 1994.

Much more was accomplished in the 1990s. As shown in Fig. 1, the numbers of reported cases of dracunculiasis have been reduced by almost 97%, to less than 100 000 in 1997, as compared to the estimated 3.2 million cases in 1986, and the nearly one million cases which were actually reported in 1989. By the end of 1997, Pakistan had been certified by WHO as free of dracunculiasis, India had halted transmission of the disease, and Yemen, the only other known affected country in Asia, had found only seven cases in the entire year. In Africa, Kenya had reported no indigenous cases since May 1994, Cameroon had only one indigenous case since September 1996, and Senegal and Chad reported only 4 and 25 cases in 1997, respectively (Fig. 2). Globally, the number of known endemic villages has been reduced from about 23 000 at the beginning of 1993, to less than 10 000 at the beginning of 1998, more than half of which are in Sudan.

Remaining challenges

Over 90% of the remaining cases of dracunculiasis are restricted to parts of only five countries (Burkina Faso, Ghana, Niger, Nigeria and Sudan). Each of these five countries presents unique difficulties, but the most serious by far is the continuing civil war in southern Sudan, where access to some of the most highly endemic foci seen anywhere in the world is severely constrained, and where the national eradication programme has not yet had any access at all to several probably endemic areas. Surveillance and control measures were less complete in Sudan in 1997 than in 1996 because of increased strife in 1997. Although the target date for global eradication of dracunculiasis was not met, our goal now is to achieve eradication as soon as possible.

Apart from the fighting in Sudan, the Dracunculiasis Eradication Programme (DEP) has suffered for many years, and continues to be plagued by opposing views held by some representatives of major partners in the campaign regarding the most appropriate strategy for implementing the programme. Some of these disagreements resulted from unrecognized differences in what was meant by "integration".

When integration means that dracunculiasis eradication activities should be among the responsibilities of all health workers in a country's established public health network, wherever possible, that is entirely appropriate. That is also exactly the approach which has been used in the DEP from the beginning — to mobilize and support otherwise underutilized members of existing health services at national, regional, and subregional levels. Those pre-existing health workers in turn supervise and support part-time village volunteers, most of whom were recruited by the DEP, because primary health care

Fig. 1. **Number of reported cases of dracunculiasis by year, 1989–97 (provisional).**

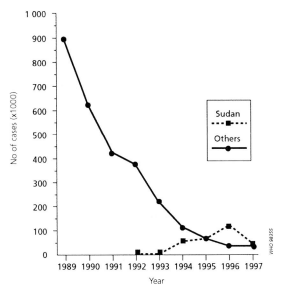

services had not reached these remote villages. Few of those health workers, and almost none of the village volunteers, are exclusively devoted to work on dracunculiasis.

In Africa, 9 of the 15 national programme coordinators of Dracunculiasis Eradication Programmes have other responsibilities in their ministries of health besides dracunculiasis eradication. In southeast Nigeria, 8 of the 10 chairmen of the state task forces for guinea-worm eradication are the state directors of public health services, in charge of all primary health care services; at the local government area (LGA) level, all of the 25 LGA coordinators for the dracunculiasis programme are local government health officials who are responsible for other health programmes. In Izzi and Ebonyi LGAs of Ebonyi State, the most endemic state in Nigeria, 100% of the 348 village level workers in the programme are unpaid volunteers, mostly farmers, not full-time "vertical guinea-worm staff", including the 4% who are community health workers with other medical responsibilities. When the DEP began in south-east Nigeria, it included all of the existing primary health care workers in endemic communities who met the programme's prerequisite criteria of residency in that village and, where possible, literacy. The situation is similar in the samples of other national DEP for which we have data: Niger, Uganda, and Mali.

When integration means using the resources which were procured for dracunculiasis eradication for other purposes, that is rarely justifiable, if at all. In my opinion when integration means turning over the active surveillance and stringent case containment which are required at the end of any eradication programme to an integrated health care system which is designed to control, not eradicate, diseases, precisely when the most intensive fo-cus on interrupting transmission is needed, that is unwise. I believe the *urgency* which is unique to eradication programmes, and the demand for excellence in implementation which that urgency requires, cannot be integrated into broader primary health care or routine health services, even when those services are working well, much less when they are not.

The rationale for the strategy of integrating control measures against dracunculiasis into other programmes appears sometimes to be motivated by a belief that the disease is not important enough to merit the intensive effort that is required to eradicate it, and by the wrong impression that control measures to eradicate dracunculiasis need to be "sustained". Aspects of these differences have been addressed recently in some publications (8–11), and I shall not repeat them here, but I would like to end this presentation by reviewing some of the indirect benefits of this eradication campaign.

Benefits of the eradication programme

Reducing the prevalence of dracunculiasis by almost 97% over the past decade is the most conspicuous achievement of the programme so far, even before eradication is fully achieved. The impact of that accomplishment on improved agricultural production alone is a major economic benefit and the World Bank, which considers an annual estimated rate of return (ERR) of ≥10% as acceptable, has calculated an ERR of 29%, based on conservative assumptions of the duration of disability from dracunculiasis (12). Indirect contributions of the programme's success so far to improved school attendance, and to the nutrition of infants and the care of toddlers in endemic households, are no less real, despite being harder to quantify.

Moreover, while realizing these accomplishments, DEP has accelerated and increased the provision of clean drinking-water by national and international agencies to thousands of endemic or formerly endemic communities, even after the Water and Sanitation Decade. It has also mobilized hundreds of communities to improve their own water supplies. In south-east Nigeria alone, for example, members of endemic villages have created more than 400 hand-dug wells in the past few years, in order to rid themselves of dracunculiasis. This is just one way that eradicating dracunculiasis has helped increase the self-reliance of some affected communities and generated ancillary benefits in the control of other waterborne diseases. The

Fig. 2. Distribution, by country, of 76 848 cases of dracunculiasis reported during 1997 (provisional).

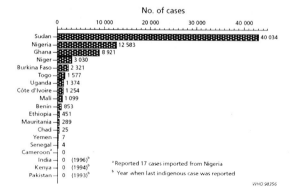

programme has also established community-based health education, village task forces, and surveillance by village volunteers in more than 15 000 remote villages (*13*). The very existence of some of those villages was previously unknown to other health workers.

The nearly 6-month long "guinea-worm cease-fire" in Sudan in 1995 also provided opportunities to treat for the first time over 100 000 persons at risk of onchocerciasis, to vaccinate over 41 000 children against measles, 35 000 against poliomyelitis, and 22 000 against tuberculosis, and to distribute more than 35 000 doses of vitamin A and treat 9000 children with oral rehydration packets, in addition to jump-starting the DEP itself in that country (*14*). And despite our sometimes divergent views, dracunculiasis eradication has succeeded as much as it has because of a broad coalition of United Nations and bilateral assistance agencies, enormous private sector contributions by the DuPont Corporation, Precision Fabrics Group, American Home Products, nongovernmental organizations, national ministries, and political leaders, all of whom have contributed to help people in endemic communities to rid themselves of this parasite.

People in these neglected communities need help. I have yet to visit an African village endemic for dracunculiasis or onchocerciasis which is suffering from too many visits by health care workers from different programmes, as some allege, requiring better integration or coordination of their health activities. The real problem is getting *any* health services to such communities. In the broad benefits it has provided and in its support of the public health staff and volunteers who are producing those benefits, one can assert with much justification that in addition to eradicating dracunculiasis, the Dracunculiasis Eradication Programme has done more to improve primary health care in endemic communities than many primary health care programmes. Primary health care was not developed in most of these communities before the DEP began, and not nearly enough is being done by health systems to build on that foundation and provide other needed services and support to the same communities once dracunculiasis is gone. I do not presume to represent the inhabitants of these neglected communities, but I do know that if I were in their place, I would prefer an excellent vertical programme to a mediocre integrated programme any day.

Acknowledgements

The assistance of Dr Eka Braide, Ms Nwando Diallo, Ms Renn Doyle, Ms Wanjira Mathai, Dr Ernesto Ruiz-Tiben and Dr James Zingeser in gathering or preparing some of the data for this paper is gratefully acknowledged.

References

1. **Hopkins DR, Ruiz-Tiben E.** Strategies for dracunculiasis eradication. *Bulletin of the World Health Organization*, 1991, **69**: 533–540.
2. **Hopkins DR.** Eradication of dracunculiasis. In: Bourne PG, ed. *Water and sanitation.* Orlando, FL, Academic Press, 1984: 93–114.
3. **Brieger WR, Watts S, Yacoob M.** Guinea worm, maternal morbidity, and child health. *Journal of tropical pediatrics*, 1989, **35**: 285–288.
4. **Tayeh A, Cairncross S.** The impact of dracunculiasis on the nutritional status of children in South Kordofan, Sudan. *Annals of tropical pediatrics*, 1996, **16**: 221–226.
5. **Hopkins DR, Foege WH.** Guinea-worm disease. *Science*, 1981, **212**: 495.
6. **World Health Organization.** Dracunculiasis surveillance. *Weekly epidemiological record*, 1982, **57**(9): 65–67.
7. **Watts SJ.** Dracunculiasis in Africa: its geographical extent, incidence and at-risk population. *American journal of tropical medicine and hygiene*, 1987, **37**: 121–127.
8. **Hopkins DR, Ruiz-Tiben E, Ruebush TK.** Dracunculiasis eradication: almost a reality. *American journal of tropical medicine and hygiene*, 1997, **57**: 252–259.
9. **Ranque P et al.** Situation actuelle de la campagne d'éradication de la dracunculose. *Médecine tropicale*, 1996, **56**: 289–296.
10. **Peries H, Cairncross S.** Global eradication of guinea worm. *Parasitology today*, 1997, **13**: 431–437.
11. **Hopkins DR.** Dracunculiasis eradication (letter). *Lancet*, 1997, **350**: 812.
12. **Kim A, Tandon A, Ruiz-Tiben E.** Cost–benefit analysis of the global dracunculiasis eradication campaign. Washington, DC, World Bank, 1997 (WB Policy Research Working Paper, No. 1835).
13. **Cairncross S, Braide EI, Bugri SZ.** Community participation in the eradication of guinea worm disease. *Acta tropica*, 1996, **61**: 121–136.
14. **World Health Organization.** Dracunculiasis and onchocerciasis — Sudan. *Weekly epidemiological record*, 1997, **72**(29): 297–301.

Perspectives from the global poliomyelitis eradication initiative

H.F. Hull,[1] C. de Quadros,[2] J. Bilous,[3] G. Oblapenko,[4] J. Andrus,[5] R. Aslanian,[6] H. Jafari,[6] J.-M. Okwo Bele,[7] & R.B. Aylward[1]

Ten years after the year 2000 target was set by the World Health Assembly, the global poliomyelitis eradication effort has made significant progress towards that goal. The success of the initiative is built on political commitment within the endemic countries. A partnership of international organizations and donor countries works to support the work of the countries. Interagency coordinating committees are used to ensure that all country needs are met and to avoid duplication of donor effort. Private sector support has greatly expanded the resources available at both the national and international level. At the programmatic level, rapid implementation of surveillance is the key to success, but the difficulty of building effective surveillance programmes is often underestimated. Mass immunization campaigns must be carefully planned with resources mobilized well in advance. Programme strategies should be simple, clear and concise. While improvements in strategy and technology should be continuously sought, changes should be introduced only after careful consideration. Careful consideration should be given in the planning phases of a disease control initiative on how the initiative can be used to support other health initiatives.

Introduction

The target to eradicate poliomyelitis by the year 2000 was set by a World Health Assembly resolution in 1988, which specified that global eradication was to be achieved within the Expanded Programme on Immunization (EPI) and within the context of strengthening primary health care (1). Since that target was set, significant progress has been achieved. However, global poliomyelitis eradication can be achieved on time only if the necessary political support and financial resources are secured. While success is not yet assured, the lessons learned during the past 10 years are relevant to the planning of future eradication initiatives. This article summarizes the perspectives from experiences with the poliomyelitis initiative in the hope that other diseases can be eradicated in the most efficient manner possible.

Strategies for poliomyelitis eradication

WHO, building on the initial successes in the Americas, defined four principle strategies for global poliomyelitis eradication: high routine immunization coverage — countries should achieve 90% immunization coverage in all districts by the year 2000; national immunization days (NIDs) — during these mass campaigns, all children aged <5 years, irrespective of their prior immunization status, should receive two doses of oral poliovirus vaccine (OPV) in rounds spaced approximately 1 month apart; surveillance for acute flaccid paralysis (AFP) — all AFP cases must be reported with clinical, epidemiological and laboratory investigation; and mopping-up immunization — house-to-house immunization campaigns should be conducted in high-risk areas identified through disease surveillance. These strategies have been discussed in detail elsewhere (2, 3).

Once wild poliovirus transmission has been interrupted, eradication must be certified by the Global Commission for the Certification of Poliomyelitis Eradication, which first met in 1995. Under the auspices of this commission, national committees are convened in all countries to collect evidence conclusively demonstrating that poliomyelitis has been eradicated. The certification process focuses primarily on the performance of the surveillance system, but also reviews information on the performance of the immunization system and documentation of preparedness to control any imported cases that may occur. Although each country must provide

[1] World Health Organization, Geneva, Switzerland.

[2] Pan American Health Organization, Washington, DC, USA.

[3] WHO Regional Office for the Western Pacific, Manila, Philippines.

[4] WHO Regional Office for Europe, Copenhagen, Denmark.

[5] WHO Regional Office for South-East-Asia, New Delhi, India.

[6] WHO Regional Office for the Eastern Mediterranean, Alexandria, Egypt.

[7] World Health Organization, Harare, Zimbabwe.

individual data, certification is on a WHO regional basis.

Progress in implementing strategies

Routine coverage with three doses of OPV worldwide has remained above 80% since 1990. Coverage is lowest in the African Region, where 12 countries are unable to immunize even 50% of infants born. As of March 1998, at least one round of NIDs had been conducted in all polio-endemic countries with the exception of the Democratic Republic of the Congo, Liberia, Sierra Leone, and Somalia. In 1997, more than 450 million children were immunized during NIDs in 80 countries worldwide. AFP surveillance has been implemented in 142 countries. Ten polio-endemic countries did not have national AFP surveillance as of March 1998. The rate of AFP cases reported is substantially below the target of 1 per 100000 annually in the African Region, where AFP surveillance is in the early phases of implementation. In the South-East Asia Region, surveillance is improving rapidly, following the posting of a large cadre of surveillance medical officers in India.

Disease incidence and challenges

The number of poliomyelitis cases reported to WHO declined by 88% between 1988 (35252 cases) and 1996 (4074 cases). As of April 1998, 3376 cases were reported for 1997 (4). However, reporting is incomplete and the final total for 1997 will approach 4000 cases. Poliomyelitis eradication was certified in the Americas in 1994, the last case being reported from Peru in September 1991 (5). At the time of writing, one year had elapsed since the last case of poliomyelitis was reported from the WHO Western Pacific Region. In the European Region, six virologically confirmed cases were reported in 1997, all from south-eastern Turkey. West and central Africa remain heavily endemic, with the Democratic Republic of the Congo and Nigeria serving as major reservoirs of wild poliovirus. South Asia is the other major global reservoir with Afghanistan, Bangladesh, India, Nepal and Pakistan remaining heavily endemic. Wild poliovirus, type 2, was identified in 1997 from only three countries — Afghanistan, India and Pakistan.

The progress achieved proves that existing technology and the WHO-recommended strategies are sufficient to eradicate poliomyelitis worldwide. The challenges that remain, however, are significant. Eradicating the disease in the remaining endemic countries will be particularly difficult because of their relative poverty, poor health infrastructure, difficult geography, dispersed populations, and ongoing armed conflict. In the most difficult countries, a substantial part of the cost of eradication must come from external sources. WHO estimates that in excess of US$ 1000 million of funds from international sources will need to be spent in the period 1998–2005 to stop wild poliovirus transmission and then certify global eradication. Mobilizing these resources and maintaining the political commitment to complete the work in the face of declining incidence are the major challenges that face the initiative. Additional challenges are the containment of laboratory strains of wild poliovirus and reaching consensus on a strategy for stopping immunization after eradication.

Lessons for future eradication initiatives

Progress towards poliomyelitis eradication has been rapid in the last 10 years, faster than some would have predicted. Within that progress, however, are both successes and failures. Just as smallpox eradication served as the foundation for poliomyelitis eradication, the successes and failures of the latter offer lessons for future eradication and elimination initiatives.

The single most important factor in the continuing success of poliomyelitis eradication is political commitment within the endemic countries. Eradication activities are conducted by the countries with the assistance of the international community. In the Americas, 80% of the cost of eradication was borne by the countries (6), while in China and Indonesia, that proportion was over 90%. The financial and human resources required for poliomyelitis eradication are, however, normally beyond the capacity of the ministry of health. Successful mass immunization campaigns require multisectoral cooperation with the involvement of the ministries of finance, transport, information, women's affairs and religious affairs, among others. The military often provides necessary transport and communication facilities. Achieving this level of intersectoral support usually requires the involvement of the head of state. Fortunately, visible and successful immunization campaigns are politically attractive and bring home the message that good health is good politics. For poliomyelitis eradication to succeed in heavily endemic countries, political commitment must be sustained for a period of at last 3–5 years.

However, eradication cannot be achieved in most polio-endemic countries without the assistance of the international community. Partnerships must be forged to ensure that sufficient resources are made available to the endemic countries. Global poliomyelitis eradication is possible because of the partnership of the governments of the endemic countries with WHO, UNICEF, Rotary International, AUSAID, CIDA, DANIDA, DFID, USAID and the governments of Japan, Norway and other countries; CDC and JICA provided critical technical support. The building of a successful coalition takes time. Each organization brings its particular strengths, and understanding the culture of each organization is vital.

Partnership is made manifest through Interagency Coordination Committees (ICCs), particularly at the national and regional level. Regular meetings of the ICC partners and representatives of the governments review the human and financial requirements for the eradication activities. The function of the ICCs is to ensure that all needs are met without duplication of effort. Partnership is also very much in evidence at annual meetings of the Global and Regional Technical Consultative Groups, during which technical staff and representatives of partner organizations meet to review progress and recommend changes in technical policy. Transparency regarding changes in programme policy facilitates the funding process.

Although the majority of financial support for poliomyelitis eradication has come from governments, significant support from the private sector has clearly accelerated the initiative. The most visible example is Rotary International, which by the end of the initiative, would have contributed more that US$ 400 million in private funds and millions of hours of volunteer time. Additional private sector support has come from businesses which paid for advertising, provided transportation, procured local commodities, and provided meals for vaccinators in the field. Individual volunteers have supported NIDs through social mobilization, transport of vaccine and vaccination staff, and free service at immunization posts. The eradication initiative has also benefited from the advocacy efforts of Rotarians and other influential persons who mobilized political support and financial resources in both endemic and polio-free countries.

The theme of partnership also extends to the area of intercountry and interregional cooperation. Microbial agents do not respect international boundaries. Since border areas are often poorly served by many government services including health, one solution to cross-border transmission has been multi-country NIDs; operation MECACAR is one such example, in which 19 countries coordinated their NIDs and immunized 60 million children (7). Specific cross-border immunization campaigns have been conducted where migratory populations have been an important reservoir. Rapid exchange of epidemiological information across international borders and interregional boundaries is vital.

Accelerated development of reliable surveillance is vital to the success of the initiative (8). For example, several countries that had apparently stopped poliovirus transmission did not have surveillance data to demonstrate that this was the case. As a result, NIDs continued for several years more than was, perhaps, necessary. In other countries, transmission of wild polioviruses might have been interrupted sooner if surveillance data had been available to identify high-risk populations. Since the cost of surveillance is less than a tenth of the total cost of poliomyelitis eradication, rapid development of surveillance systems should be seen not just as a necessity, but also as a cost-saving measure.

The difficulty of establishing surveillance is often underestimated. Surveillance is much less visible than immunization campaigns and is often perceived as a lower priority. Delays in developing surveillance systems result from a number of factors. Establishing AFP reporting and building the capacity for case investigation typically takes several years. Physicians and other clinical health care personnel who are likely to see cases must be trained to the rationale and methods for AFP surveillance. Active surveillance through weekly visits to health facilities that are most likely to see such cases are usually required. Case investigation teams must be trained and provided with transport and travel allowances. Electronic communication does not substitute for the face-to-face meetings required to build effective teams. In the laboratory network, training laboratory staff and retaining them is a continuing challenge. A stock of reagents and disposable supplies must be maintained for all network laboratories. Although every attempt was made to use existing, functional virology laboratories, capital equipment purchases are often necessary. Assessing equipment needs, securing funds, procuring, and shipping are all time-consuming activities.

Monitoring the quality of surveillance through the use of standard, internationally comparable performance indicators is central to success. Reporting must be complete and timely to permit effective action. As poliomyelitis incidence decreases, reporting of AFP cases becomes increasingly important because these could possibly be poliomyelitis. Surveillance indicators were developed to monitor the effectiveness of the surveillance system. The most important of these are the AFP rate, the percentage of AFP cases with two adequate stool specimens, and the timeliness and completeness of reporting by district. Supervisory visits to the field are necessary and often reveal problems and solutions that could not be appreciated from the central level. Laboratory performance must also be measured in a similar, but more comprehensive manner. Laboratories must be formally accredited and regularly demonstrate their proficiency with blinded samples. Useful laboratory process indicators are the percent of specimens with non-polio enteroviruses and the percent of specimens analysed within 28 days of receipt of the sample.

The availability of simple and safe technology has been central to the successful implementation of poliomyelitis eradication strategies. Because OPV is administered orally, many countries have used trained volunteers as vaccinators (9). This approach greatly expands the work force available to conduct NIDs, increases the speed with which NIDs can be conducted, and raises the coverage achieved. The ultimate volunteer vaccinator is the head of state. The opportunity for high-level politicians to be filmed immunizing children both increases the political support for the initiative and sends a powerful message to government and health workers alike.

Successful immunization campaigns require adequate planning and budgeting for logistics and social mobilization, extending down to the district level. Campaigns conducted without sufficient lead time and the necessary planning and resource mobilization have been substandard. With sufficient forward planning and coordination with donors, multiyear grants were made in some countries, permitting technical staff to focus on programme implementation rather than fundraising. In planning, one must also recognize that the cost of bringing together the child and the intervention greatly exceeds that of the intervention itself. The cost per child per year for two doses of OPV is approximately US$ 0.20. However, the average cost of training, social mobilization and operations to deliver that vaccine is US$ 0.80 per child. In the most difficult countries, operational costs can rise to US$ 3 per child immunized.

Technological changes that simplify logistics and reduce costs produce the greatest advantages to the initiative. For smallpox, these were the jet injector and then the bifurcated needle. One important technological advance for the poliomyelitis eradication initiative is the individual vaccine vial monitor (VVM), a thermosensitive marker which changes colour when exposed to heat. VVMs allow a vaccinator with minimal training to tell at a glance if a vaccine vial has been exposed to excessive heat. They increase confidence that the vaccine is potent at the time of administration and permit OPV to be taken out of the cold chain. The genetically engineered murine L20B cell line is another new technology that is currently being introduced into network laboratories. This change is expected to reduce the workload and markedly increase the reliability of cell culture for the identification of polioviruses. Technology, which was proposed but not incorporated into the eradication initiative, include using IPV and stabilizing OPV with deuterium oxide. These technical changes provided only marginal improvements in efficiency and/or could not be made available in time to make a significant impact. The search for improved technology should continue as the initiative progresses, but efforts should promote quantum leaps rather than incremental gains.

Similarly, strategies must be continuously reviewed to improve efficiency and, where possible, make changes that reduce cost and simplify logistics. Changes in strategy that have been adopted by the poliomyelitis eradication initiative include the following: an emphasis on hospital-based, active surveillance to increase AFP case detection; elimination of routine collection of specimens from case-contacts (benefits were small while overloading laboratory capacity); and a de-emphasis of localized outbreak response immunization (scientific review indicated minimal impact on virus transmission). Strategists must keep in mind that frequent or unnecessary changes in strategy produce confusion. Complexity must also be avoided since activities are conducted by field staff in developing countries. Accordingly, strategies must be simple and consistent and changed only after careful consideration.

While other health initiatives may benefit from the eradication initiative, requests to combine other activities with the eradication activities must be considered carefully. In the course of the poliomyelitis eradication initiative, for example, vitamin A capsules have been administered during NIDs, while measles vaccine and tetanus toxoid have been administered to selected high-risk populations, and dracunculiasis searches have been conducted in a major guinea-worm reservoir. However, caution must be exercised so that the objectives of the eradication activity are not compromised. Thorough planning is necessary so that adequate human and financial resources are secured for the additional tasks.

Recently there has been considerable debate over the impact of poliomyelitis eradication activities on primary health care (10). The Taylor Commission reviewed the issues in the Americas after eradication was achieved there (11); the report was supportive, but the sociological approach taken provided insufficient documentation to resolve the debate. Another study has been started, but the results are unlikely to be available until the final phases of the initiative. Although poliomyelitis eradication has increased immunization coverage and improved the quality of services in countries with poorly developed immunization programmes and sustained the level of coverage in countries with good immunization services, this information has not been systematically collected or disseminated. Future initiatives should include early documentation of all the benefits including reduced morbidity and mortality. It may, therefore, be useful to consider during the planning phases the benefits to other health systems from eradication activities.

Conclusion

While the last case of poliomyelitis is still several years in the future, the success of the global poliomyelitis eradication initiative can serve as a model for future disease eradication and elimination initiatives. As strategies for those initiatives are being defined and consensus to move forward is built, political support and funding for the final and most difficult phase of eradication must continue. Since failure of the poliomyelitis (or dracunculiasis) eradication initiatives would jeopardize support for any future eradication initiative, significant challenges must be met. The global poliomyelitis eradication initiative remains on track and global certification is expected shortly after the turn of the century. When that occurs, every child in every country will be free of the risk of poliomyelitis forever.

References

1. *Global eradication of poliomyelitis by the year 2000.* Geneva, 1988 (resolution WHA41.28). In: *Handbook of resolutions and decisions of the World Health Assembly and the Executive Board*, vol. III, third ed. (1985–1992). Geneva, World Health Organization, 1993.

2. **de Quadros CA et al.** The eradication of poliomyelitis: progress in the Americas. *Pediatric infectious diseases*, 1991, **10**: 222–229.

3. **Hull HF et al.** Paralytic poliomyelitis: seasoned strategies, disappearing disease. *Lancet*, 1994, **343**: 1331–1337.

4. **Expanded Programme on Immunization.** Progress towards global poliomyelitis eradication, 1988–1997. *Weekly epidemiological record*, 1998, **73**(22): 161–168.

5. **Robbins FC, de Quados CA.** Certification of the eradication of indigenous transmission of wild poliovirus in the Americas. *Journal of infectious diseases*, 1997, **175** (Suppl. 1): S281–S285.

6. **de Quadros CA, Nogueira AC, Olivé JM.** Roles for public and private sectors in eradication programs. In: Dowdle WR, Hopkins DR, eds. *The eradication of infectious diseases: report of the Dahlem Workshop on the Eradication of Infectious Diseases*. Chichester, John Wiley & Sons 1998: 117–124.

7. **Expanded Programme on Immunization (EPI).** Update: mass vaccination with oral poliovirus vaccine — Asia and Europe, 1996. *Weekly epidemiological record*, 1996, **71**(44): 329–332.

8. **Andrus JK, de Quadros CA, Olivé JM.** The surveillance challenge: final stages of eradication of poliomyelitis in the Americas. In: CDC Surveillance Summaries. *Morbidity and mortality weekly report*, 1992, **41**(SS-1): 21–26.

9. **Banerjee K, Andrus JK, Hlady G.** Conquering poliomyelitis in India. *Lancet*, 1997, **349**: 1630.

10. **Aylward RB et al.** Disease eradication initiatives and general health services: ensuring common principles lead to mutual benefits. In: Dowdle WR, Hopkins DR, eds. *The eradication of infectious diseases: report of the Dahlem Workshop on the Eradication of Infectious Diseases*. Chichester, John Wiley & Sons 1998: 61–74.

11. **Taylor Commission.** *The impact of the Expanded Program on Immunization and the Polio Eradication Initiative on health systems in the Americas.* Washington, DC, Pan American Health Organization, 1995.

Measles eradication: experience in the Americas

C.A. de Quadros,[1] B.S. Hersh,[2] A.C. Nogueira,[2] P.A. Carrasco,[2]
& C.M. da Silveira[2]

In 1994, the Ministers of Health from the Region of the Americas targeted measles for eradication from the Western Hemisphere by the year 2000. To achieve this goal, the Pan American Health Organization (PAHO) developed an enhanced measles eradication strategy. First, a one-time-only "catch-up" measles vaccination campaign is conducted among children aged 9 months to 14 years. Efforts are then made to vaccinate through routine health services ("keep-up") at least 95% of each newborn cohort at 12 months of age. Finally, to assure high population immunity among preschool-aged children, indiscriminate "follow-up" measles vaccination campaigns are conducted approximately every 4 years. These vaccination activities are accompanied by improvements in measles surveillance, including the laboratory testing of suspected measles cases.

The implementation of the PAHO strategy has resulted in a marked reduction in measles incidence in all countries of the Americas. Indeed, in 1996 the all-time regional record low of 2109 measles cases was reported. There was a relative resurgence of measles in 1997 with over 20000 cases, due to a large measles outbreak among infants, preschool-aged children and young adults in São Paulo, Brazil. Contributing factors for this outbreak included: low routine infant vaccination coverage, failure to conduct a "follow-up" campaign, presence of susceptible young adults, and the importation of measles virus, apparently from Europe.

PAHO's strategy has been effective in interrupting measles virus circulation. This experience demonstrates that global measles eradication is an achievable goal using currently available measles vaccines.

Introduction

In 1994, the countries of the Region of the Americas established the goal of eliminating measles from the Western Hemisphere by the year 2000 (1). Measles is one of the most highly infectious diseases, and in the prevaccine era, essentially everyone eventually acquired measles infection, usually as a very young child. Humans are the only reservoir for measles infection, although some other primates, such as monkeys, can be infected. The patient is most infectious during the prodromal phase of the disease before the onset of symptoms such as fever and rash. Communicability decreases rapidly after the appearance of rash (2).

Live attenuated measles vaccine, first licensed for use in the USA in 1963, was in widespread use by the late 1970s (3). Immunization with this vaccine has been demonstrated to be protective for over 20 years, but immunity following vaccination is thought to be life-long (4). Vaccine efficacy has been shown to be 90–95%. Because of interference of maternal antibodies, vaccine efficacy increases steadily after 6 months of age, reaching its maximum plateau of 95–98% at 12–15 months of age.

By 1982, virtually all countries in the world had incorporated measles vaccine into their routine vaccination schedules and, since then, coverage has increased substantially. By 1990, the estimated overall global coverage for children by 2 years of age was approximately 70%. Before the introduction of measles vaccine, epidemics characteristically tended to recur every 2–3 years in most densely populous areas, but with the widespread use of measles vaccine, the interval between outbreaks has lengthened (5, 6) and an increase in the average age of infection is observed. In the developing countries which recently introduced the vaccine and have not yet achieved high immunization coverage, measles remains endemic with most cases occurring in young children and infants (7). WHO has estimated that 40 million measles cases, with 1 million deaths, are still occurring annually in the world.

PAHO measles eradication strategy

The Pan American Health Organization (PAHO) recommends a strategy that aims to interrupt rapidly measles transmission by initially conducting a one-time-only mass campaign targeting all children aged 9 months to 14 years and to maintain interruption of transmission by sustaining high population immu-

[1] Pan American Health Organization, Washington, DC, USA.
[2] Special Program for Vaccines and Immunization, Pan American Health Organization, Washington, DC, USA.

nity through vaccination of infants at routine health services facilities, supplemented by periodic mass campaigns conducted approximately every 4 years, targeting all 1–4-year-olds, regardless of previous vaccination status. "Fever and rash" surveillance and measles virus surveillance are other key elements of the strategy (8).

The initial "catch-up" measles vaccination campaign is conducted during periods of low measles transmission. All children aged 9 months to 14 years, irrespective of vaccination history or reported history of measles infection, are immunized with measles vaccine within a very short period of time, usually one week to one month. These campaigns result in a rapid increase in population immunity and, if high enough coverage is achieved, measles transmission is interrupted. After a catch-up campaign has been conducted, there may still remain pockets of susceptible children. To detect these, a post-catch-up campaign evaluation is conducted and special vaccination (mop-up) activities are carried out in such areas to increase their level of coverage.

After the initial catch-up campaign and mop-up operations, routine immunization services (keep-up) should ensure that all new birth cohorts of children are vaccinated with a dose of measles vaccine at 12–15 months of age. However, there will inevitably be an accumulation of susceptible preschool-aged children over time. Two major factors contribute to the accumulation of susceptibles. First, measles vaccine is not 100% effective, thus leaving some children unprotected despite vaccination. Second, measles vaccination coverage for each birth cohort will fall short of 100%, however effective the programme.

Thus, the PAHO strategy calls for periodic vaccination campaigns to be conducted among preschool-aged children (children <5 years of age). This is recommended whenever the estimated number of susceptible preschool-aged children approaches the size of an average birth cohort. In the Americas it is recommended that such follow-up campaigns be conducted every 4 years.

A sensitive surveillance system is essential for a measles elimination programme. This includes the notification and timely investigation of infants and children with suspected measles. Serological testing for anti-measles IgM antibodies in blood specimens obtained from suspected cases is used to confirm or rule out measles virus infection. A confirmed measles case must either have serological confirmation or an epidemiological link to another laboratory-confirmed measles case. Laboratory sequencing of the measles virus genome from isolates can help to determine geographical sources of outbreaks and identify pathways of transmission.

Since 1991, all PAHO Member countries, with

the exception of the USA, have conducted catch-up measles vaccination campaigns (Table 1) and most countries have already conducted at least one follow-up campaign.

Summary of impact

In the Region of the Americas, reported cases have decreased markedly and the majority of countries have reported a 99% reduction in measles incidence compared to the prevaccine era. Several countries have already interrupted transmission. In Cuba, after the catch-up campaign conducted in 1987 and a follow-up campaign conducted in 1991, fewer than 20 confirmed measles cases were reported annually between 1989 and 1992, with the last serologically confirmed case occurring in June 1993 (9).

Other countries in the Region of the Americas in which transmission apparently has been interrupted include the English-speaking Caribbean, which conducted its catch-up measles vaccination campaign during May 1991. Between September 1991 and March 1997, only two confirmed measles cases were reported in the English-speaking Caribbean — in Barbados (one acquired the infection in New York City, and no source of infection could be found for the other). No secondary spread of infection occurred (10). After Chile conducted its catch-up campaign during 1992, only one case was discovered in 1992 (imported from Peru) and one in 1993 (imported from Venezuela). No further spread occurred until a recent importation from Brazil, in 1997. Transmission in this outbreak has now been interrupted.

During 1996 the Region of the Americas recorded an all-time low of only 2109 confirmed measles cases (Fig. 1). In 1997, however, there was a relative resurgence of the disease in Brazil. Up to 31 January 1998, a total of 78 033 suspected measles cases was reported from the countries of the Americas. One third of these (26 722 (34.2%)) have been confirmed; and 25 559 of these were reported from Brazil alone which, with Canada (580 confirmed cases), accounted for 97.8% of the total confirmed cases in the region. Other countries reporting measles cases in 1997 included Guadeloupe (128 cases), USA (127 cases), Paraguay (124 cases), Argentina (58 cases), Chile (47 cases), and Costa Rica (14 cases). The outbreaks in Argentina, Chile, Costa Rica, Chile and Paraguay originated from importations from Brazil, and the Guadeloupe epidemic was due to an importation from metropolitan France in late 1996 (11). This island had not implemented PAHO's recommended measles eradication strategy.

Table 1: **Countries conducting catch-up and follow-up campaigns, 1987–97** .

Region Country/territory	Campaign 1–14 years (Catch-up)		Average routine coverage 1994–96 (Keep-up)	Campaign 1–4 years (Follow-up)	
	Year	Coverage (%)		Year	Coverage (%)
Andean					
Bolivia	1994	98	90	—[a]	—
Colombia	1993	96	93	1995	90
Ecuador	1994	100	70	—[a]	—
Peru	1992	75	87	1995	97
Venezuela	1994	100	75	—[a]	—
Brazil					
Brazil	1992	96	80	1995	77
Central America					
Belize	1993	82	82	1995	85
Costa Rica	1993	75	90	—[a]	—
El Salvador	1993	96	89	1996	82
Guatemala	1993	85	73	1996	60
Honduras	1993	96	91	1996	85
Nicaragua	1993	94	81	1996	97
Panama	1993	88	86	1996	94
English-speaking Caribbean					
Anguilla	1991	99	97	1996	100
Antigua and Barbuda	1991	96	95	1996	92
Bahamas	1991	87	91	1997	78
Barbados	1991	96	98	1996	91
Cayman Islands	1991	85	92	—[a]	—
Dominica	1991	95	95	1996	100
Grenada	1991	98	89	1996	81
Guyana	1991	94	84	1996	90
Jamaica	1991	71	87	1995/6	95
Montserrat	1991	100	100	1996	100
St. Kitts and Nevis	1991	98	100	1996	100
St. Lucia	1991	97	94	1996	85
St. Vincent and Grenadines	1991	97	100	1995	84
Suriname	—[a]	—	75	—[a]	—
Trinidad and Tobago	1991	90	88	1997	96
Turks and Caicos	1991	91	98	1996	95
Virgin Islands (British)	1991	86	100	1996	90
Latin Caribbean					
Cuba	1987	98	100	1993	99
Dominican Republic	1993	77	84	—[a]	—
Haiti	1994	94	28	—[a]	—
Mexico					
Mexico	1993	88	91	—[a]	—
Southern Cone					
Argentina	1993	97	98	—[a]	—
Chile	1992	99	94	1996	100
Paraguay	1995	70	78	—[a]	—
Uruguay	1994	95	88	—[a]	—

[a] Follow-up campaign was to be conducted before writing of this paper.

In the USA, over half of the cases originated from importations from Europe and Asia. Spread from importations has been limited and the largest outbreak in 1997 was only 8 cases. In 1995 and 1996, there were no measles importations from Latin America or the Caribbean into the USA (*12*). In 1997, however, there were 5 confirmed imported cases from Brazil (*13*) (Fig. 2).

The majority of cases from Brazil have been reported from São Paulo State, the only state in the country which did not conduct a follow-up vaccination campaign in 1995 (*13*). To date, over 20 000 cases have been confirmed in this outbreak, with most cases in the city of São Paulo. Over 50% of cases occurred in young adults aged 20–29 years. The highest age-specific incidences are in infants, young

Fig. 1. **Reported measles cases among 1-year-old children in the Americas, 1980–97** (source: PAHO/WHO).

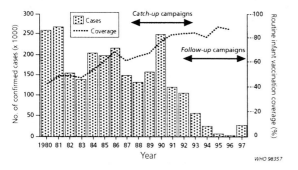

Fig. 2. **Importation of measles from Latin American countries and the Caribbean into the USA, 1990–97** (source: CDC, Atlanta, GA, USA).

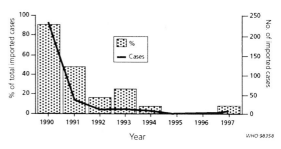

adults aged 20–29 years, and children aged 1–4 years, respectively. To date, 20 measles-related deaths have been reported, most in infants aged <1 year. An investigation of measles cases in adults found that the majority were occurring among young adults who were members of certain risk-groups including men who recently migrated to cities from rural areas in the north-east of the country to work in construction projects, other manual labourers, students, health care workers, persons working in the tourist industry, and military recruits (14).

Measles virus has been isolated from several patients from this outbreak and the genomic sequencing of these isolates revealed that the virus circulating in São Paulo is virtually identical to that currently circulating in Western Europe, which strongly suggests importation from the latter area (14). The São Paulo outbreak is waning after implementation of an aggressive outbreak response, which included a follow-up campaign targeting all children aged 1–4 years, selective mop-up vaccination in schools, and vaccination of young adult members of groups at high-risk for measles (14).

Until 1997, the English-speaking Caribbean had not reported a single confirmed case of measles in a period of over 5 years (13). However, in 1997 two laboratory-confirmed measles cases were detected. The first was reported from the Bahamas. The patient, a young adult, had rash onset in March 1997. The direct source of transmission was not identified, but it is strongly suspected that the patient contracted measles from a tourist. A search, involving a review of over 80 000 diagnoses from health facilities in the country, was made to identify any additional cases of measles. The second case was reported from Trinidad and Tobago. It occurred in a young adult Italian sailor who had rash onset in April. The

patient had acquired measles in Italy. A specimen was collected and found to be positive for measles IgM at the measles laboratory of the Caribbean Epidemiology Centre (CAREC). No spread of cases was identified despite careful investigation.

Discussion

While the resurgence of measles in the Americas during 1997 represents a major increase compared to cases reported in 1996, these cases represent only about 10% of those reported in 1990. Nevertheless, important lessons can be learned from this experience. First, the lack of a timely follow-up vaccination campaign in São Paulo, in 1995, for children aged 1–4 years, combined with low routine measles vaccination coverage (keep-up) among infants using a 2-dose schedule, allowed for a rapid and dangerous accumulation of susceptible children. Second, the presence of large numbers of young adults who escaped both natural measles infection and measles vaccination increased the risk of a measles outbreak. Third, measles virus was imported into São Paulo, probably from Europe. Finally, the high population density in São Paulo facilitated contact between persons infected with measles and susceptible persons.

Measles case surveillance combined with molecular epidemiological data suggest that the countries of the Region of the Americas are constantly being challenged by imported measles virus from other regions of the world where measles remains endemic (15). During 1997, 27 separate importations of measles virus were detected from Europe, 18 from Asia, and 2 from Africa (Fig. 3) which resulted in measles transmission (13). These data, however,

Fig. 3. **Measles importations into the Region of the Americas, 1997** (source: SVI/PAHO and CDC, Atlanta, GA, USA).

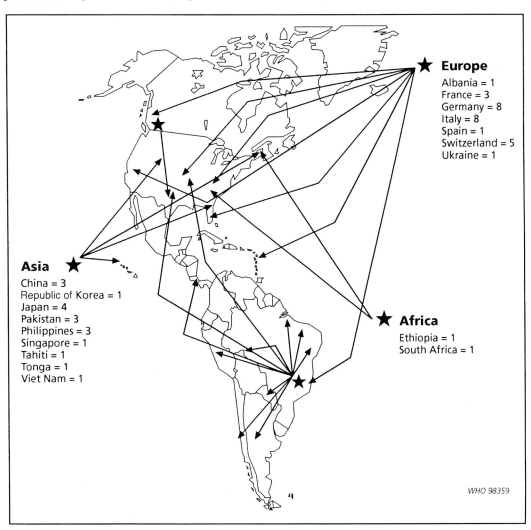

probably severely underestimate the true number of measles importations since many imported cases may not seek medical care and do not result in further transmission.

The outbreaks in Brazil, Canada and other countries of the region suggest that there may be a significant number of young adults who remain susceptible to the disease. For practical purposes, persons born before 1960 in most countries of the Region of the Americas can be assumed to have been exposed to naturally circulating measles virus, and thus be immune to the disease. Therefore, the

overwhelming majority of adults are already immune, and most susceptible young adults are at very low risk of being exposed to measles virus.

Mass campaigns among young adults are not recommended. However, experience has shown that certain institutional settings (e.g. colleges and universities, military barracks, health care facilities, large factories, and prisons) can facilitate measles transmission, if measles virus is introduced to such populations. In addition to persons living or working in these settings, adolescents and young adults who travel to countries with endemic measles transmission are at increased risk of being exposed to and contracting measles. To prevent the occurrence of measles outbreaks among adolescents and young adults, efforts are needed to ensure measles immunity in these potentially high-risk groups and persons travelling to measles-endemic countries.

The measles experience of 1997 clearly demonstrates that there are two major challenges to the region's measles eradication goal by the year 2000. First, the countries of the Region of the Americas need to maintain the highest population immunity possible in infants and children, and to target vaccination to adolescents and young adults who are at highest risk for being exposed to measles virus. Second, increased efforts are needed in other regions of the world to improve measles control and to decrease the number of exported measles cases to the Region of the Americas. As long as measles virus circulates anywhere in the world, the Region of the Americas will remain at risk for measles. The successful achievement of the measles elimination goal in the Region of the Americas will require full implementation of PAHO's recommended immunization strategy in all countries of the region and improved measles control/elimination in other regions of the world, especially Europe and Asia, with the ultimate goal of global eradication of the measles virus (16).

References

1. **Pan American Health Organization.** Measles elimination by the year 2000. *EPI Newsletter*, 1994, **16**: 1–2.
2. **Krugman S et al.** *Infectious diseases of children.* 8th edition. St. Louis, Missouri, C.V. Mosby Company, 1985.
3. **Krugman S et al.** Studies with a further attenuated live measles-virus vaccine. *Pediatrics*, 1963, **31**: 919–928.
4. **Markowitz LE et al.** Duration of measles vaccine-induced immunity. *Pediatric infectious disease journal*, 1990, **9**: 101–110.
5. **Fine PEM, Clarkson JA.** Measles in England and Wales — I. An analysis of factors underlying seasonal patterns. *International journal of epidemiology*, 1982, **11**: 5–14.
6. **Mclean AR, Anderson RM.** Measles in developing countries, Part I. Epidemiological parameters and patterns. *Epidemiology and infection*, 1988, **100**: 111–133.
7. **Clements CG et al.** The epidemiology of measles. *World health statistics quarterly*, 1992, **45**: 285–291.
8. **de Quadros CA et al.** Measles elimination in the Americas: evolving strategies. *Journal of the American Medical Association*, 1996, **275**: 224–229.
9. **Galindo MA et al.** The eradication of measles from Cuba. *Pan American journal of public health* (in press).
10. **Hospedales CJ.** Update on elimination of measles in the Caribbean. *West Indian medical journal*, 1992, **41**: 43–44.
11. **Pan American Health Organization.** Update: recent measles outbreaks in the Americas. *EPI newsletter*, 1997, **19**: 3.
12. **Centers for Disease Control.** Measles — United States, 1996, and the interruption of indigenous transmission. *Morbidity and mortality weekly report*, 1997, **46**: 242–246.
13. **Pan American Health Organization.** Measles in the Americas, 1997. *EPI newsletter*, 1997, **19**: 1–3.
14. **Pan American Health Organization.** Update: São Paulo measles outbreak. *EPI newsletter*, 1998, **20**(1): 5–6.
15. **Rota JS et al.** Molecular epidemiology of measles virus: identification of pathways of transmission and implications for measles elimination. *Journal of infectious diseases*, 1996, **173**: 32–37.
16. **Centers for Disease Control.** Measles eradication: recommendations from a meeting co-sponsored by the World Health Organization, the Pan American Health Organization and CDC. *Morbidity and mortality weekly report*, 1997, **46** (RR-11): 1–31.

CANDIDATE DISEASES FOR ELIMINATION OR ERADICATION

Introduction: identification of candidate diseases

The conference participants' consideration of candidate diseases and conditions for elimination or eradication included overviews for each of the four basic disease categories — noninfectious conditions, and bacterial, parasitic, and viral diseases. The conditions and diseases highlighted in the overviews were identified during the spring of 1997 through a survey of persons invited to the conference.

The survey form was sent to 167 invited participants and 109 responded. The form enumerated conditions or diseases in each of the four basic categories and provided spaces for listing additional conditions. Each recipient was asked to rank, for each group, up to four conditions to be considered during the conference. Although the set of conditions reflected a strong level of agreement, it was not intended to constrain workgroup decisions from deleting some or adding others.

Following the overview, the workgroups received a charge and a framework for addressing important issues and candidate conditions. There were two primary goals for each of the four condition-specific workgroups (a fifth workgroup addressed the topic of sustainable health development): first, to agree on the set of specific candidate conditions to be addressed by the group; and second, for each of the agreed-upon candidate conditions, by using the fact sheets and additional information, to deliberate and specify basic considerations, including essential facilitating factors (e.g. research and technologies, political/organizational will, and partnerships), key strategies to accomplish the objective(s), research needs, and relevant conclusions and recommendations regarding the elimination/eradication of the condition. Each workgroup was led by two co-chairs, and each group had a principal rapporteur. Each full workgroup was required to achieve a high level of agreement on the core elements and recommendations.

Candidate noninfectious disease conditions

D. Alnwick[1]

Important micronutrient deficiencies in at-risk populations can be addressed simultaneously with program-matically cost-effective results. Because of the interaction between many micronutrients, this would also be biologically effective.

With adequate investment and political support, the chances of eliminating iodine deficiency as a problem in women of reproductive age and young children and of eliminating vitamin A deficiency as a problem in young children in the future are high. To eliminate iron deficiency and folic-acid-dependent neural tube defects (FADNTDs) in low-income populations, a new set of approaches will have to be developed. These same approaches, if successful, could be used to tackle other important micronutrient deficiencies.

Introduction

Before the conference, a large number of health policy experts were asked to rank nine noninfectious disease conditions in the order of how feasible their elimination appeared to them, as well as to suggest other potential candidates. Only one additional condition was proposed: protein–energy malnutrition. Their responses showed that the four top-ranking candidates for elimination were iodine-deficiency disorders (IDDs), vitamin A deficiency, iron-deficiency anaemia, and folic-acid-dependent neural tube defects (FADNTDs). This article reviews the feasibility of eliminating these four conditions, which are caused by an inadequate dietary intake of one or more micronutrients. Our increasing understanding of the interaction between nutritional status and infection suggests that large-scale efforts to eradicate particular infectious diseases will probably be greatly strengthened if efforts are made simultaneously to eliminate specific micronutrient deficiencies.

Candidate conditions for elimination

Ten noninfectious disease conditions were proposed as potentially eliminable. The top four (mentioned above) are due to inadequate intake of a specific nutrient; the fifth, lead intoxication, is due to the excess dietary intake of an antinutrient; and the seventh, fluoride deficiency, is due to the inadequate intake of an ion that is arguably a nutrient.

It is surprising that vitamin D deficiency was not identified as a candidate for potential elimination. There is substantial evidence to indicate that vitamin D deficiency is still common in young children and women of child-bearing age in developing countries, particularly (but not exclusively) among people living north of latitude 30° (1). There is also evidence suggesting that the consequences of inadequate vitamin D intake on child health and survival are more damaging than believed so far (2).

Zinc deficiency was also not proposed as a candidate condition for elimination. This was perhaps because the respondents did not believe there was adequate consensus on its importance or on the feasibility of interventions. It is likely, however, that zinc deficiency is at least as prevalent as iron deficiency, that its harmful consequences for child survival and development are as important as those of the latter, and that a modification of interventions to reduce the prevalence of iron deficiency could simultaneously, and at little additional cost, also reduce the prevalence of zinc deficiency (3).

Women during the earliest period of pregnancy are the principal target group for both the elimination of IDDs and the prevention of FADNTDs. Improving the intake of both iodine and folate will also benefit other population groups, particularly young children and adolescents, and, in the case of folate, adults at risk of coronary heart disease (4). Traditionally, pregnant women have been the primary focus of efforts to prevent iron-deficiency anaemia, but increasing emphasis is being placed both on ensuring adequate iron status in women prior to pregnancy and on reducing iron-deficiency anaemia in young children (5).

Vitamin A deficiency has until recently been considered to be a problem almost exclusively of young children. However, there is growing recognition that in some countries, particularly in South Asia, a substantial proportion of pregnant women also suffer from vitamin A deficiency and that the implications for maternal health are as severe and important as those relating to child health and survival (6).

[1] Chief, Health Section, United Nations Children's Fund (UNICEF), New York City, New York, USA.

Need for concerted global action

Micronutrient deficiencies contribute substantially to the high young-child mortality, poor maternal health, and high prevalence of childhood disability in developing countries (7, 8). Although the control or elimination of noninfectious, micronutrient deficiency diseases in one country or region could certainly be achieved independently of actions elsewhere, there are strong reasons to support coordinated international action to eliminate micronutrient deficiencies in parallel with global efforts to eradicate infectious diseases. These include the exchange of experiences and technologies between countries, and the creation of a favourable international environment which will make action by any particular national government less risky. For example, when the intervention is food fortification, harmonization of standards between countries will help ensure that fortification does not become an impediment to trade between countries.

Eliminating micronutrient deficiencies will facilitate the elimination or eradication of some infectious diseases

It is becoming increasingly clear that the high prevalence of general malnutrition and of some specific micronutrient deficiencies in developing countries, particularly among young children, increases the incidence, severity, duration and other characteristics of many of the infectious diseases that are considered to be candidates for elimination or eradication. Consequently, efforts to improve nutrition and eliminate micronutrient deficiencies should be seen as an important part of disease control, elimination, and eradication efforts. In addition, many of the infectious diseases being considered as candidates for elimination or eradication also contribute to malnutrition and micronutrient deficiency through reduced absorption of nutrients, increased utilization and loss of nutrients, and anorexia. Elimination or eradication of these infectious diseases will therefore improve nutrition.

The relationship between vitamin A deficiency, the immune system, and infectious diseases is perhaps the best understood of all micronutrient deficiency–infection interactions. In the last decade, epidemiological, immunological and molecular studies have yielded substantial evidence for a central role for vitamin A in ensuring optimum immune function (9). Measles is more severe and more likely to be life-threatening in children who are vitamin-A deficient (10). A study from Ghana (11) suggests that the incidence of measles may also be higher in vitamin-A-deficient children. The antibody response to measles vaccine, given in a single dose at 9 months of age, was greater in children who received vitamin A supplements in Guinea-Bissau (12, 13). A depressed immune response to tetanus immunization in vitamin-A-deficient children was demonstrated in Indonesia (14).

The goal of global elimination of IDDs was adopted at the 1990 World Summit for Children principally because it was recognized that a substantial amount of mild and moderate mental impairment in children could be avoided if all women received an adequate iodine intake during pregnancy. There is recent evidence that, in areas of moderate and severe iodine deficiency, increasing the iodine intake of the population through supplements or the addition of iodine to irrigation water substantially reduces infant mortality, presumably by improving immune function (15).

There is some evidence that the incidence and severity of malaria infection is lower in young children supplemented with zinc or vitamin A in areas where these micronutrient deficiencies are common (3). Micronutrient deficiencies may play a role in other parasitic diseases. For example, zinc supplementation reduced the intensity of *Schistosoma mansoni* reinfections in Zimbabwe (16). There appear to have been no randomized controlled trials to determine the effect of improving micronutrient status on other parasitic infections, but animal studies suggest that vitamin A deficiency may increase the filariasis worm load and zinc deficiency may increase ascaris parasite loads (17, 18). There is also evidence of a possible causal association between low serum retinol levels, low vegetable consumption, and risk of hepatocellular carcinoma, which is the main reason why viral hepatitis B is being considered as a possible candidate for eradication (19).

The observation that selenium and vitamin E deficiencies can cause a normally benign coxsackievirus in mice to mutate and become virulent, suggests that poor nutrition, in addition to compromising the immune system of the host, may also permanently influence the genetic make-up of the pathogen itself (20, 21). If this observation is confirmed to be of significance in human populations, it will further change our understanding of the interaction of nutrition and infection.

Interventions to eliminate micronutrient deficiencies

There are four major interventions that are likely to be effective in successfully eliminating — within the next decade — the four candidate micronutrient deficiencies in young children, women of child-bearing age, and pregnant women. These interventions are as follows: 1) the direct administration of a large "bolus" dose of a nutrient at infrequent intervals by a trained health worker to individuals in the target population at a health facility or during special mass campaigns akin to national immunization days; 2) the supply to families of lower-dose micronutrient supplements to be taken by at-risk members daily, weekly, or possibly monthly, over a period of several months or years – these supplements might be provided through health facilities and schools or distributed through commercial channels at an affordable price; 3) the fortification of a "staple food" that is consumed in relatively constant amounts by the target groups; and 4) the manufacture and distribution (through commercial or other channels) of a specially designed fortified food, beverage, or food additive containing the desired micronutrients — this product would be marketed or distributed so that the at-risk population had sufficiently increased intake of the candidate micronutrients. Table 1 shows a summary of recent experience with each of these four groups of interventions for each of the priority candidate conditions.

Large, single doses of micronutrients given infrequently

The success achieved in reducing the prevalence of vitamin A deficiency in young children has hinged on the fact that relatively large doses the vitamin can be stored in the liver and released, as needed, over a period of up to 6 months. Liver stores can be built up by administering large oral doses of retinol to young children once every 4–6 months. This has proved to be a highly effective, low-cost way of improving the vitamin A status of tens of millions of young children. It is estimated that about 50% of young children at risk of vitamin A deficiency, in countries that recognize the problem, currently receive at least one high dose of vitamin A (22).

High-dose iodine supplements have been provided to women of child-bearing age through injections or through oral solutions of iodine in vegetable oil. However, with the increasing recognition that salt iodization is the method of choice for eliminating iodine deficiency almost everywhere, the need for large, periodic doses of iodine will in future be limited to populations who cannot be provided with iodized salt.

Table 1: **Summary of interventions to correct iodine, vitamin A, iron and folate deficiencies**

Nutrient	Intervention category			
	Large periodic doses with immunization-like contacts	Low-dose supplements taken at home	Fortification of staple food	Provision of low-bulk, processed food, beverage or fortificant for home use, which contains multiple micronutrients
Iodine	Oral and injectable doses, given once every year; available, safe and effective; useful only where salt iodization is impossible or for "mopping up"	Feasible, but not widely tested; limited need due to effectiveness of salt iodization	Salt iodization proven to be widely feasible and effective	Very limited trials in El Salvador and United Republic of Tanzania
Vitamin A	High oral doses very effective in young children and postpartum women, extensively used	Feasible, but very limited experience with use	Sugar in Central America and Philippines; wheat or maize feasible	Ditto
Iron	History of use of injectable iron; effective in women; safety questioned in children	Effective, considerable experience; low cost; formulations for young children not yet available; growing evidence of effectiveness of weekly supplements	Long history of wheat fortification, little data on impact	Ditto
Folate	Not feasible	As for iron, but effectiveness of weekly supplements unknown	Recent introduction of cereal fortification in the USA and Australia	Ditto

Injectable iron compounds were successfully used to control iron-deficiency anaemia in pregnant women in Sri Lanka, but this method has not been widely used elsewhere. Iron-deficiency anaemia in young children was controlled with injectable iron in some industrialized countries, but this method was discontinued following reports of adverse reactions.

Low-dose micronutrient supplements, taken frequently at home

In 48 developing countries there are national policies for routinely providing supplies of iron or combined iron/folate supplements to pregnant women, to be taken daily at home. In 29 of these countries it was estimated that at least 50% of pregnant women received supplements (UNICEF survey, 1997). There has recently been extensive debate on the effectiveness of daily iron supplementation programmes, focused on issues that reduced the impact of these programmes, such as inadequate logistics and supply, poor compliance due to side-effects, and inadequate absorption.

In some industrialized countries, the majority of pregnant women are advised to take multivitamin and mineral supplements, which have not been widely used in developing countries. In parts of Europe where iodine deficiency is a concern and where iodized salt is not widely consumed, pregnant women are generally advised to consume daily supplement tablets containing iodine.

A combined daily supplement containing folate, vitamin A, and iron could certainly be provided to large populations of women of child-bearing age in the form of a small daily tablet. Other essential micronutrients could easily be added to this tablet at very low additional cost including, for example, zinc, selenium, vitamin D, and the B group vitamins.

Although there is still no consensus on the relative effectiveness of daily versus weekly doses of iron in pregnancy, there is agreement that efforts to treat and prevent iron-deficiency anaemia before women become pregnant is desirable, and that long courses with small doses of iron are preferable to short courses of high doses.

Weekly supplements containing both iron and vitamin A could be provided to reproductive-age women and would probably be effective in improving iron and vitamin A status. Vitamin D could also be effectively added to such a weekly tablet. As it is not known whether folic acid or zinc status could be improved by the use of a weekly dose of these micronutrients, given as part of a combined weekly supplement, this is an important area for research.

Fortification of widely consumed foods and salt

Fortification of food and salt has enormous potential advantages. Public expenditure and the additional burden on the health sector can be kept to a minimum, especially as costs are generally low and can be easily passed on to the consumer. The requirements for successful fortification programmes are well documented (24). There are, however, few options for fortification of staple foods in the developing countries which have the greatest prevalence of micronutrient deficiencies. The four foods or condiments which are most amenable to fortification in low-income countries are, in decreasing order of importance, salt, sugar, vegetable oil, and cereal flour.

Salt has proven to be the vehicle of choice for delivering iodine to populations in North America and much of Europe for the last 60 years or more. Over the last 10 years, the salt industry in almost all developing countries has been approached by governments, international agencies, and other concerned parties and encouraged or required to fortify with iodine all salt sold for human and animal consumption. These efforts have been extremely successful. It is currently estimated that over 50% of all salt consumed in developing countries is now fortified, compared with less than 10% in 1990.

The possibility of adding other "target" nutrients to salt needs to be seriously considered. There is some experience with fortifying salt with iron (25), and a controlled trial of salt fortified with both iodine and iron is under way in Ghana. There are considerable technical obstacles to fortifying salt with reactive iron. If the present trials are successful, wider production of double-fortified salt may be possible. However, because of the additives and more complex processing required, the cost of double-fortified salt is likely to be substantially greater than that of salt fortified with iodine alone, and it is unlikely that many governments of developing countries will in the near future be able to require all salt to be double fortified.

The recent unsuccessful experience in attempting to support the large-scale fortification of the flavour enhancer monosodium glutamate (MSG) with vitamin A in Indonesia suggests that the large-scale fortification of salt with vitamin A is not feasible. There is currently no information on the feasibility of fortifying salt with folic acid or zinc. Such studies are urgently needed.

Fortification of "special" foods

A potentially promising approach to tackling multiple micronutrient deficiencies in at-risk populations is the production and promotion of a "special" food; for example, a flavoured drink mixture, or a flavoured powder that could be stirred into a child's food. A pilot study of such an intervention for young children and pregnant women — using a low-cost drink mix powder — has recently been completed in the United Republic of Tanzania with UNICEF support, and a study of the effectiveness of a fortified-powder sachet, which is added to a child's complementary food, is under way in Nicaragua, supported by the USAID OMNI Project.

Dietary improvement

Dietary improvement, though critically important in itself, is unlikely to secure rapid progress in eliminating the priority micronutrient candidate conditions; hence its exclusion from the above short-list of priority interventions. Education to modify the composition of diets (independent of the two interventions discussed above) will have little impact on eliminating iodine deficiency, since foods naturally rich in iodine tend to be rare and expensive, or on eliminating FADNTDs. Education to increase the consumption of animal muscle or offal-based food, to increase the intake of iron absorption promoters such as vitamin C, and to reduce the intake of inhibitors such as tannin, will make a modest contribution to reducing iron deficiency. Education to increase the consumption by target groups of food containing pro-vitamin A carotenoid and animal products rich in retinol will also contribute to eliminating vitamin A deficiency, but the experience with present interventions suggests that this will rarely, if ever, be sufficient to move most members of a population group from deficiency to adequacy in a short period. The inclusion of vitamin A and iron deficiency elimination goals into the nutrition objectives of countries' agriculture and food policies must be encouraged, with the long-term objective that appropriate policies will help to sustain the elimination of these deficiencies, hence allowing some of the interventions listed above to be phased out by around 2020. Ongoing efforts to increase the vitamin A, iron, and zinc availability in staple foods through plant breeding need to be strongly encouraged, but for another decade or more are unlikely to substantially contribute to the goal of eliminating iron or vitamin A deficiency.

Conclusions

Elimination of iodine deficiency

The iodization of edible salt has proved to be a highly effective intervention in almost every country,

and must be continued. Quality control and monitoring need to be strengthened. If the present rate of increase in the use of iodized salt continues, it is likely that within the next few years iodine deficiency will be eliminated as a public health problem in most countries. A major challenge ahead is to maintain political support for salt iodization programmes in countries where these programmes have succeeded in reducing the prevalence of visible signs of deficiency, such as goitre. Additional interventions, such as the iodization of irrigation water or the use of supplements, will be needed in areas where it is very difficult to iodize salt.

Elimination of vitamin A deficiency in children

Expanded use of high-dose vitamin A supplements will substantially reduce the prevalence of vitamin A deficiency in young children. All countries where vitamin A deficiency exists as a public health problem, and all countries with high under-5-year-old mortality rates should promote routine use of high-dose vitamin A supplements, provided once every 4–6 months to all young children over the age of 6 months, generally, or on national immunization days. In countries where cereal flour or sugar is widely consumed in relatively constant amounts, the fortification of these foods with vitamin A is likely to help reduce vitamin A deficiency and anaemia among both young children and reproductive-age women.

Elimination of iron-deficiency anaemia, FADNTDs, and vitamin A deficiency in women

Fortification of staple foods with iron and folic acid will probably sharply reduce anaemia and FADNTDs in the limited number of developing countries where centrally processed staples are widely consumed. Routine micronutrient supplementation of reproductive-age women with supplements of folic acid, iron, and vitamin A, together with other micronutrients, would probably greatly contribute to the elimination of all three of these conditions. A combined daily supplement would be effective, but would be costly and compliance might be difficult to ensure. A weekly supplement may also be effective — and would be cheaper — but more research is needed on the effectiveness of weekly doses and on compliance in unsupervised settings.

Iron-deficiency anaemia in young children

Infants in all countries are at high risk of iron deficiency after 6 months of age because of their high iron needs associated with rapid growth. Low-birth-weight infants, who are born with lower iron stores, may be at high risk of deficiency at an even earlier age. Where iron-fortified infant foods are not widely and regularly consumed by young children, infants should receive iron supplements in the first year of life. Continued supplementation may be needed for another year if family diets are lacking in available iron.

References

1. **Alnwick D.** Review of recent progress in tackling micronutrient malnutrition in developing countries. Should vitamin D be higher on the agenda? In: Norman AW et al., eds. *Vitamin D: chemistry, biology and clinical applications of the steroid hormone.* Proceedings of the Tenth Workshop on Vitamin D, Strasbourg, France, 24–29 May 1997. Riverside, CA, University of California, 1997.

2. **Muhe L.** Case-control study of the role of nutritional rickets in the risk of developing pneumonia in Ethiopian children. *Lancet*, 1997, **349**: 1801–1804.

3. *Zinc for Child Health: Report of a meeting, Baltimore, MD, 17–19 November 1996.* Baltimone, MD, Johns Hopkins School of Public Health (Child Health Research Project Special Report, June 1997, vol. 1, no. 1).

4. **Collaboration HLT.** Lowering blood homocysteine with folic-acid-based supplements: meta-analysis of randomised trials. *British medical journal*, 1998, **316**: 894–898.

5. **Viteri F.** Prevention of iron deficiency. In: Howson C et al., eds. *Prevention of micronutrient deficiencies: tools for policymakers and public health workers.* Washington, DC, National Academy Press, 1998.

6. Vitamin A supplements save pregnant women's lives. *State of the world's children 1998.* New York, UNICEF, 1998: 12–13.

7. *State of the world's children 1998.* New York, UNICEF, 1998.

8. **Csete J.** Malnutrition and disability. *Child health dialogue*, 1997, Issue 7. London, AHRTAG.

9. **Semba R.** Effect of vitamin A supplementation on immunoglobulin G subclass responses to tetanus toxoid in children. *Clinical journal of diagnostic laboratory immunology*, 1994, **1**(2): 172–175.

10. **Sommer A.** Vitamin A, infectious disease, and childhood mortality. *Journal of infectious diseases*, 1993, **167**: 1003–1007.

11. **Dollimore N.** Measles incidence, case fatality, and delayed mortality in children with or without vitamin A supplementation in rural Ghana. *American journal of epidemiology*, 1997, **146**: 646–654.

12. **Benn CS.** Randomised trial of effect of vitamin A supplementation on antibody response to measles vaccine in Guinea-Bissau, West Africa. *Lancet*, 1997, **350**: 101–105.

13. Vindication of policy of vitamin A with measles vaccination. *Lancet*, 1997, **350**: 81–82.

14. **Semba RD.** Depressed immune response to tetanus in children with vitamin A deficiency. *Journal of nutrition*, 1992, **122**: 101–107.

15. **DeLong R.** Effect on infant mortality of iodination of irrigation water in a severely iodine-deficient area of China. *Lancet*, 1997, **350**: 771–773.

16. **Friis H.** Serum concentrations of micronutrients in relation to schistosomiasis and indicators of infection: a cross-sectional study among rural Zimbabwean schoolchildren. *European journal of clinical nutrition*, 1996, **50**: 386–391.

17. **Sturchler D.** Retinol deficiency and *Dipetalonema vitea* infection in the hamster. *Journal of helminthology*, 1985, **59**: 201–210.

18. **Laubach HE.** Effect of dietary zinc on larval burdens, tissue eosinophil numbers, and lysophospholipase activity of *Ascaris suum* infected mice. *Acta tropica*, 1990, **47**: 205–211.

19. **Yu MW.** Vegetable consumption, serum retinol level, and risk of hepatocellular carcinoma. *Cancer research*, 1995, **55**: 1301–1305.

20. **Beck M.** Increased virulence of coxsackievirus B3 in mice due to vitamin E or selenium deficiency. *Journal of nutrition*, 1997, **127**: 996S–970S.

21. **Levander O.** Nutrition and newly emerging viral diseases: an overview. *Journal of nutrition*, 1997, **127**: 948S–950S.

22. **Alnwick D.** Combating micronutrient deficiencies: problems and perspectives. *Proceedings of the Nutrition Society*, 1998, **57**: 137–147.

23. **Lotfi M et al.** *Micronutrient fortification of foods: current practices, research and opportunities.* The Micronutrient Initiative, Ottawa, 1996.

24. **Ranganathan S.** Large-scale production of salt fortified with iodine and iron. *Food and nutrition bulletin*, 1996, **17**: 73–78.

Candidate bacterial conditions

M.L. Cohen[1]

This article provides background information on bacterial diseases and discusses those that are candidates for elimination or eradication. Only one disease, neonatal tetanus, is a strong candidate for elimination. Others, including Haemophilus influenzae b *infection, leprosy, diphtheria, pertussis, tuberculosis, meningococcal disease, congenital syphilis, trachoma and syphilis are important causes of morbidity and mortality in industrialized and developing countries. For all these diseases, eradication/elimination is not likely because of the characteristics of the disease and limitations in the interventions.*

Background

In 1900, infectious diseases — especially bacterial diseases — were the leading cause of morbidity and mortality, and diseases such as tuberculosis and pneumococcal infection were called the "Captain of all these men of death". A series of factors that began in the 16th and 17th centuries and extended into the 20th century greatly influenced the frequency of infectious diseases. These factors included improvements in hygiene and sanitation, better housing and nutrition, and safer food and water; the technological advances of the 20th century include use of vaccines and antibiotics. It is important to emphasize that, particularly for bacterial diseases, any reduction in their frequency is multifactorial and related to both specific and nonspecific changes. For example, examination of the estimated and reported mortality for tuberculosis in England from 1700 to 1920 shows a peak around 1770 at a rate of 700 per 100 000 — carrying a nearly 1% chance per year of dying of tuberculosis. By 1920, the mortality rate had decreased to less than 50 per 100 000. This decline preceded the introduction of BCG and anti-tuberculosis chemotherapy. Thus, factors such as improvements in nutrition, decreased crowding, and better hygiene and sanitation were major contributors to the reduction in the incidence of tuberculosis. As we approach the 21st century, bacterial diseases and infectious diseases in general are no longer the leading causes of death in the developed world, except for certain conditions (e.g. heart disease) which may have a significant infectious etiology, as is currently being discussed. Globally, however, the perspective is different. For example, in 1992, almost 20 million deaths were caused by infectious and parasitic diseases, which WHO estimates to have been the leading cause of death worldwide. Bacterial disease (e.g. tuberculosis and other respiratory and diarrhoeal diseases of bacterial etiology) accounted for more than half of these deaths.

Bacterial diseases are not static but include newly emerging diseases, re-emerging diseases that were once thought to be conquered, and diseases that show changes of antimicrobial resistance. For example, in the last two decades, bacterial diseases have been newly recognized, including Legionnaires' disease, toxic shock syndrome, Lyme disease, campylobacteriosis, *Escherichia coli* 0157:H7 infections, helicobacter infections associated with peptic ulcer disease, and *Bartonella* infections associated with cat scratch disease. Cholera is an example of a re-emerging disease in the Western hemisphere which, since 1991, has caused over a million cases and 10 000 deaths. Other diseases, such as meningococcal infections, *Salmonella enteritidis* infections associated with shelleggs, foodborne listeriosis, and tuberculosis have increased in frequency, in some instances in both the industrialized and developing world. Antimicrobial resistance, once thought to be primarily a problem of hospital-acquired infections, is also a particular problem among community-acquired infections. In the hospital, there are strains of enterococci and tuberculosis that are essentially untreatable with antimicrobials, and strains of *Staphylococcus aureus* that have become relatively resistant to vancomycin — the last effective antimicrobial for many of these strains. In the community, drug-resistant infections with pneumococci, salmonella, shigella, and gonococci have become important public health problems. For example, strains of *Shigella dysenteriae* 1A in parts of the developing world have become resistant to almost every oral antimicrobial agent. Many strains of multidrug-resistant pneumococci are only susceptible to vancomycin.

One final point involves the often unexpected consequences of changes that either intentionally or unintentionally affect the frequency of bacterial dis-

[1] Director, Division of Bacterial and Mycotic Diseases, National Center for Infectious Diseases, Centers for Disease Control and Prevention, Atlanta, GA 30333, USA.

eases. In the latter part of the 19th century and into the 20th century, efforts were made to improve hygiene and sanitation in many parts of the developed world. In Germany, for example, with increases in the number of homes in Frankfurt-am-Main that were connected to sewers and water mains, the death rate from typhoid fever rapidly decreased. However, an unexpected impact of such improvements in hygiene and sanitation in the developed world resulted in postponement or prevention of the exposure of many parts of the population to poliomyelitis, creating a population susceptible to epidemics and paralytic disease at a later age. Thus, efforts to eliminate or eradicate one disease may have important implications for another.

Candidate conditions

Based on the responses from the conference participants to identify potential candidates for elimination or eradication, only one bacterial disease — neonatal tetanus — was felt to be a strong candidate for elimination. There was relatively little difference in support for other bacterial diseases, including *Haemophilus influenzae* b infection, leprosy, diphtheria, pertussis, tuberculosis, meningococcal disease, congenital syphilis, trachoma, and syphilis. The low level for most bacterial diseases relates, in part, to various deficiencies in the criteria for elimination or eradication. For many of these diseases, there are either inadequate diagnostic methods or inadequate interventions, or there are reservoirs that persist in the environment or animal populations. Thus, for most bacterial diseases, eradication is not feasible and elimination is extremely complicated.

Neonatal tetanus — the one potential candidate for elimination — is a devastating illness caused by infection with *Clostridium tetani*, usually of the umbilical stump. The case-fatality ratio for this infection is greater than 80% and it ranks second only to measles as a cause of childhood mortality among the vaccine-preventable diseases that are included in the Expanded Programme on Immunization. It is estimated that annually there are over 490 000 deaths from neonatal tetanus, accounting for a global mortality rate of 6.5 per 1000 live births. Effective interventions include vaccination coverage with two doses of tetanus toxoid among women of childbearing age in high-risk areas. This approach, coupled with efforts to promote clean delivery and core care practices, as well as evaluation of the role of topical antimicrobial agents, provides a potential to eliminate this disease. Elimination goals have been set by WHO and, between 1980

and 1995, the number of developing countries that eliminated neonatal tetanus increased from 38 to 97.

Haemophilus influenzae is also an important cause of global morbidity and mortality, causing meningitis, pneumonia, and septicaemia. In the USA, prior to the introduction of conjugate vaccines, an estimated 1 in 200 children were affected by age 5 years. At present, the estimates of the global burden of disease range from 380 000 to 600 000 deaths annually in children aged <5 years. The potential for elimination or eradication of this disease has been supported by the introduction of effective conjugate vaccines. These vaccines have led to a significant reduction in the incidence of invasive *Haemophilus influenzae* type B disease in the developed world (e.g. in the USA, > 95% reduction). In addition, in several industrialized countries, the vaccine has led to significant reduction in the carriage rate of this organism. Even though these achievements suggest that effective use of the vaccine may lead to global eradication of related disease, several barriers persist, including its high cost and the lack of data on both the effectiveness and the impact on carriage in developing countries compared with the developed world.

Leprosy (Hansen's disease) is an ancient problem whose control has long been complicated by an incubation period that can range from 2 to 40 years. Although the disease appears to have low infectivity, there remain questions about the occurrence of transmission, including the relative importance of person-to-person and environmental transmission. The current prevalence of the disease is greater than 1.1 million, a substantial decline from the 10–12 million in recent years. None the less, 500 000 new cases occur annually, predominantly in 55 countries throughout the world. Perhaps the greatest impact on this disease has been the demonstrated effectiveness that multidrug therapy is curative. In contrast to the previous life-long therapy of patients infected with its causative agent, *Mycobacterium leprae*, multidrug regimens are curative within 6–12 months. Although these regimens have raised optimism for elimination of leprosy, there are, as with any chronic multidrug therapy, issues of compliance and microbial resistance.

Diphtheria had been under good control in most developed countries until the early 1990s when it resurged, particularly in the Newly Independent States of the former Soviet Union. Although the specific explanation for this resurgence is unclear, continued circulation of toxigenic strains and waning immunity in adults have been postulated as possible explanations. Interventions include an inexpensive and safe toxoid and a pattern of seasonal transmission that presents the opportunity for interruption of transmission. Pertussis is also an important cause of global morbidity and mortality accounting annually for 39 million cases and 355 000 deaths. Although intervention is part of routine infant immunization programmes, immunization does not prevent carriage or circulation of the strain in the community and current schedules do not provide immunization for adults. Thus, waning immunity in adults, continuing carriage, infection and disease limit the effectiveness of interventions. In addition, diagnostic tests are of limited effectiveness and the lack of surrogates for protection complicate the development of new vaccines. Congenital syphilis is another candidate for elimination. There is an estimated 70% probability of transmission from an infected pregnant woman to the fetus. Over 900 000 infected pregnancies occur globally each year, resulting in 360 000 fetal or perinatal deaths and the births of 270 000 infants with serious or permanent impairment. The intervention strategy involves testing of all pregnant women for syphilis and the treatment of all positives with penicillin. Penicillin remains an excellent intervention tool since it is both inexpensive and the spirochaete has not developed resistance. Most of the issues that could affect elimination of this disease are operational.

Conclusion

Bacterial diseases remain an important cause of morbidity and mortality in both the developed and the developing world. The emergence of new and re-emergence of old bacterial diseases, and the development of antimicrobial resistance pose substantive challenges to public health. For most bacterial diseases, eradication is not likely and any plans for elimination are complicated by the characteristics of the disease and limitations in intervention.

Candidate parasitic diseases

K. Behbehani[1]

This paper discusses five parasitic diseases: American trypanosomiasis (Chagas disease), dracunculiasis, lymphatic filariasis, onchocerciasis and schistosomiasis. The available technology and health infrastructures in developing countries permit the eradication of dracunculiasis and the elimination of lymphatic filariasis due to Wuchereria bancrofti. *Blindness due to onchocerciasis and transmission of this disease will be prevented in eleven West African countries; transmission of Chagas disease will be interrupted. A well-coordinated international effort is required to ensure that scarce resources are not wasted, efforts are not duplicated, and planned national programmes are well supported.*

Introduction

The Division of Control of Tropical Diseases (CTD) in WHO has global responsibility for African trypanosomiasis, Chagas disease, dracunculiasis (guinea-worm disease), foodborne trematode infections, intestinal parasitic infections, leishmaniasis, lymphatic filariasis, malaria, onchocerciasis and schistosomiasis. National programmes to combat these diseases are supported by WHO, in many instances in collaboration with other international agencies, development aid agencies, nongovernmental organizations, and industry. The mission of CTD, working closely with the WHO Regional Offices, is to provide support to country activities, to promote, advocate and coordinate tropical disease control with the aim of improving the health status of individual communities and populations, and to contribute to social and economic development.

This paper discusses five of the diseases listed above: Chagas disease, dracunculiasis, lymphatic filariasis, onchocerciasis and schistosomiasis. Four of these have been targeted for global elimination by the World Health Assembly, the objectives being the interruption of transmission of Chagas disease by the year 2010; the eradication of dracunculiasis by 2008; the elimination of lymphatic filariasis by 2020; and the elimination of onchocerciasis as a public health problem in 11 West African countries by 2002.

Criteria for establishing elimination programmes

Technical feasibility is the criterion for changing from control of infection to an objective of elimination or interruption of transmission. This requires that the disease has been adequately researched in terms of the causative organism, clinical impact, management, treatment and epidemiology. The change is facilitated by a breakthrough in the form of a new strategy and/or tool that can effectively and rapidly reduce the incidence of infection and disease using the infrastructures in place.

Public health strategy

Disease elimination or eradication programmes have to fit within the existing public health strategies. The essential public health functions in each country should include major parasitic disease problems as an integral and coherent part of the "Renewal of Health for All" process led by WHO.

Determinants of success or failure

The definitions of success and failure are never very clear and these terms tend to be used to promote different points of view. Perhaps the criteria for success or failure should be spelled out from the very beginning. There are, however, many factors that determine success or failure, and the major issues are discussed below.

- A good surveillance system and sensitive response mechanism are essential to monitor progress, detect epidemics and programme deficiencies, and take remedial action.

- Research is needed to provide the scientific basis upon which to make programme adjustments — operational research to answer questions that will improve programme implementation and management, and basic research to evaluate new tools and determine the conditions under which they will provide optimum results.

- Both political will and commitment are absolutely essential and these should be demonstrated by

[1] Director, Division of Control of Tropical Diseases, World Health Organization, 1211 Geneva 27, Switzerland.

provision of the necessary resources to implement well-planned programmes with clear strategies and in-built evaluation procedures.

- Basic training and continuing education at all levels are crucial, and supervision should be seen as a part of the educational process. The right mix of highly trained specialists and generalists and systems for motivation are important.

- Community participation and coordinated national and international action are required to avoid duplication of effort and to maximize impact.

Chagas disease

The objective is the interruption of vectorial and transfusional transmission in the Americas, by the year 2010, of the blood-borne parasite *Trypanosoma cruzi* which causes Chagas disease. Natural transmission occurs through the bite of triatomine bugs and iatrogenically through blood transfusion. The strategy, therefore, is to eliminate both vectorial and transfusional transmission by the household application of insecticides and through blood bank screening.

There are 16–18 million infected persons in Central and South America and 100 million people at risk. Currently, human infection of young age groups has been reduced by 68% over the last 6 years in the Southern Cone countries (Argentina, Brazil, Bolivia, Chile, Paraguay and Uruguay). In 1997, Uruguay had eliminated the vector *Triatoma infestans*, demonstrating that elimination of transmission is a feasible goal.

A similar initiative for the Andean countries (Colombia, Ecuador, Peru, and Venezuela) was launched in February 1997 with preparation of detailed plans of action and budget for 1998 to 2001. It is foreseen that interruption of vectorial and transfusional transmission will be achieved in these countries by 2005. Similar efforts for the Central American countries were launched in October 1997; it is foreseen that transmission will be interrupted by 2010.

Dracunculiasis

The disease is caused by a parasitic worm *Dracunculus medinensis* (guinea worm). The infection is acquired by humans through drinking water containing infected cyclops. This minute crustacean becomes infected by ingestion of the larvae of *Dracunculus* which are released into water when an infected person steps into it to relieve the pain caused by the emerging worm. The emergence of the adult worm through the skin, usually from the legs and feet, approximately one year after the individual concerned drank unsafe water, is extremely painful, causing fever, nausea and vomiting, and disabling the person for months.

There are 100 million people still at risk of infection. In 1997 alone, approximately 70000 cases were reported, compared to the estimated 10 million individuals infected per annum before the inception of the eradication programme. This drastic reduction is the result of the efforts made jointly by the countries with WHO, UNICEF, CDC, Global 2000 and a multitude of other NGOs and industry. Although there are no specific drugs to treat or prevent infection, the recommended strategy aims at case containment of infected individuals, community-based surveillance, and provision of safe drinking-water through the distribution and use of cloth filters.

Lymphatic filariasis

Lymphatic filariasis, often referred to as elephantiasis, causes profound lymphoedema, genital and renal involvement, and secondary bacterial infections, and can result in disfiguring enlargement of the limbs, breasts, and genitalia. It is endemic in 73 countries, where 120 million people are infected. Worldwide it is estimated that there are 25 million cases of genital disease and 15 million cases of lymphoedema/elephantiasis. The disease is caused by a blood-borne infection with the parasitic worms *Wuchereria bancrofti*, *Brugia malayi*, and *B. timori*, which are transmitted by various mosquito species. Humans are the only definitive host for *W. bancrofti*, which accounts for 90% of infections. For *B. malayi* and *B. timori*, which account for the remaining 10%, a number of other animals may harbour the parasites. However, the epidemiological role of this in relation to transmission is thought to be small.

Epidemiologically it has been shown that, where hygiene and environmental improvements predominate, there can be a reduction in parasite levels to below those necessary to sustain local transmission. Introduction of simple treatment regimens can greatly hasten the interruption of transmission. Largely because of newly available and dramatically effective treatment and diagnostic tools, the outlook for filariasis control/elimination is now so positive that it has been identified as a potentially eradicable disease. WHO has therefore embarked upon the global elimination of lymphatic filariasis as a public health problem globally by the year 2020. To this end, SmithKline Beecham in December 1997 agreed to donate albendazole and support the programme until the disease has been eliminated.

Onchocerciasis

Onchocerciasis is caused by infection with the filarial worm *Onchocerca volvulus*, which is transmitted by blackflies of the genus *Simulium*, causing itching and a disfiguring skin disease, serious eye lesions, and blindness among persons in parts of tropical Africa, the Arabian peninsula, and Central and South America. Although the control of onchocerciasis by the Onchocerciasis Control Programme in West Africa has been highly successful, the disease remains endemic in 34 countries, affecting over 17 million people, 99% of whom are in Africa. At least 6.5 million people suffer severe itching or dermatitis and at least 270 000 are blind because of the worm infection.

The strategy that has been shown to be most effective is the annual single-dose treatment of affected populations with the drug ivermectin, and larviciding against the blackfly vector. In 1997, 18 million treatments were given, approximating to 25% coverage. It is possible to sustain this programme due to a drug donation programme by Merck & Co.

The policy aims at prevention of blindness and elimination of onchocerciasis as a public health and socioeconomic problem throughout Africa and the Americas, and interruption of onchocerciasis transmission in selected foci. In the eleven Onchocerciasis Control Programme countries in West Africa, elimination is expected by 2002, and the participating countries are expected to maintain this. In the African Programme for Onchocerciasis Control covering the remaining endemic countries in Africa, the objective is to have established — by 2005 — effective, self-sustaining, community-based ivermectin treatment programmes which will lead to the elimination of this disease from the rest of Africa. In the Onchocerciasis Elimination Programme of the Americas, it is expected that — by 2000 — morbidity will have been reduced and blindness and other sequelae prevented, leading to the elimination of the pathological manifestations of the disease and interruption of transmission in selected foci.

Schistosomiasis

Schistosomiasis is a parasitic waterborne trematode infection causing chronic ill health and affecting the urinary or intestinal system. Intestinal schistosomiasis is caused by the flatworms or blood flukes, *Schistosoma mansoni*, *S. japonicum*, *S. mekongi* and *S. intercalatum*, while urinary schistosomiasis is caused by *S. haematobium*. People are infected by contact with water used in normal daily activities for personal or domestic hygiene and when swimming, or through occupational activities such as fishing, rice cultivation, and irrigation. The intermediate hosts are different species of snail which, when infected, release cercariae into the water which can penetrate the intact skin. In the human, it is not the worm but the eggs which cause damage to the intestine, bladder, and other organs.

The global distribution of schistosomiasis has changed significantly over the past 30 years, as a result of successful control in Asia, the Americas, North Africa, and Middle East. This success has been consistently linked to both political commitment and the implementation of a concerted control strategy. However, schistosomiasis remains endemic in 74 developing countries (600 million people at risk) and infects more that 200 million people (120 million with symptoms and 20 million suffering the severe consequences of the disease). The greatest concern is in sub-Saharan Africa, where over 80% of the cases occur.

The main intervention strategy is an integrated approach using chemotherapy, health education, the installation of wells and safe water sources and latrines, and the control of snails. Today, the global objective remains control, especially in Africa, where transmission continues to be intense. Moreover, recent environmental changes, closely linked to water resources development in previously low or nonendemic areas and increases in population densities, have led to the spread of this disease.

The rationale

It has long been realized that dracunculiasis can only be contracted by drinking water that contains infected *Cyclops*. Thus, the source of drinking-water is the crucial link in the cycle. Ever since the United Nations launched the International Drinking Water Supply and Sanitation Decade (1981–1990), the possibility of dracunculiasis eradication became a reality.

In the Southern Cone countries of South America, the vector of Chagas disease is found inside houses in close proximity to humans and control of transmission has proved to be amenable by use of insecticides, house design, and routine blood screening. In the Andean and Central American countries, the habits of the vector species are more extradomiciliary so that vector control will be more difficult and progress slower.

The decision to include lymphatic filariasis as a disease for global elimination was taken, based on advances during the last decade or two in diagnosis, clinical understanding, treatment and control of this disease, as well as the increasing political commitment by Member States. Today, interruption of transmission can be achieved by treating infected persons and by mass treatment of the population at risk. The mainstay of the elimination strategy is the use of simple, safe, inexpensive and conveniently delivered drugs that kill microfilariae and that have some effect on the adult worms.

The very successful Onchocerciasis Control Programme in West Africa was well funded and well managed. The advent of the drug ivermectin, the initiation of the Mectizan Donation Programme, the participation of the ministries of health, nongovernmental organizations, WHO and other collaborating agencies in drug distribution programmes, and rapid epidemiological assessment techniques and mapping methods have given rise to well-founded optimism. Thus, interruption of transmission in selected foci is feasible in these areas in a relatively short space of time with a combination of drug therapy and vector control. In the remaining countries of Africa and in the Americas, the programmes are at the early stage of development and implementation.

Schistosomiasis remains difficult to control because environmental changes which are taking place favour the intermediate host. Even though there has been a major decrease in prevalence and distribution of S. japonicum and S. haematobium, the bulk of transmission remains in sub-Saharan Africa. In Africa the disease is strongly linked with poverty, movement of populations, contamination of water, and agricultural practices. In this continent control remains a difficult task. The poorest countries where schistosomiasis is prevalent do not have the economic potential (national or family level) to organize and coordinate effective and sustainable disease control. Thus, schistosomiasis is not at present among those diseases listed for elimination in the next two decades.

Conclusions

The available technology and health infrastructures in developing countries permit the eradication of dracunculiasis and the elimination of lymphatic filariasis due to W. bancrofti, which will benefit present and future generations. Progress in controlling infections due to B. malayi and B. timori will depend upon future studies on the impact of the epidemiological overlap between the animal and human infection. Persons now suffering from elephantiasis will require special case management. Blindness due to onchocerciasis will be prevented and disease transmission will be interrupted in the eleven West African countries which were in the original Onchocerciasis Control Programme. Transmission of Chagas disease will also be interrupted, leaving a residue of chronic sufferers to be managed by the health services.

The lessons learned from present attempts to eradicate/eliminate/interrupt transmission of the above-mentioned four diseases and the health service systems that are strengthened in the process should contribute to the elimination/eradication of other tropical diseases in the not too distant future. The efficiency and effectiveness of programmes must be strengthened so that the gains achieved can be sustained in the long term. This will require building the capacity of health systems, education, training of health professionals, community mobilization, and information, education, and communication (IEC) activities.

Success calls for a well-coordinated international effort to ensure that scarce resources are not wasted, efforts are not duplicated, and planned national programmes are well supported. Clear priorities and a more equitable distribution of resources should be made by national governments and by international and development aid agencies and nongovernmental organizations.

Candidate viral diseases for elimination or eradication

F. Fenner[1]

This article discusses the possibilities for elimination or eradication of four viral diseases — measles, hepatitis B, rubella and yellow fever.

Introduction

The results of a preliminary survey to identify the top three or four viral diseases that could be considered as candidates for eradication or elimination resulted in the following scores (on an arbitrary scale): 185 for measles, 90 for hepatitis B, 71 for rubella, 42 for yellow fever, 27 for rabies, and 27 for mumps — with hepatitis A, rotaviral enteritis and varicella as also-rans. In view of the conclusions of the Dahlem Workshop in 1997 (1), it is surprising that yellow fever and rabies, which have animal reservoirs, were included, because these diseases cannot be candidates for either elimination or eradication, although their control could be greatly improved. The present article will deal with the first four diseases on the above list — measles, hepatitis B, rubella and yellow fever — and also briefly, mumps.

Measles

Progress on the eradication of measles, which poses a heavy disease burden (about 36 million cases and a million deaths annually) and satisfies the biological criteria that were considered essential for eradication by the Dahlem Workshop, has already been presented by de Quadros (2). The criteria are as follows:

• A specifically human disease, with no animal reservoir.

• An acute, self-limiting disease, infectious for others for only about a week; only two exceptions — inclusion body encephalitis (a rare complication occurring in immunosuppressed individuals), and subacute sclerosing panencephalitis (SSPE) (a disease of unknown etiology). In neither of these conditions is measles virus excreted or released into the environment, so that they have no epidemiological significance.

• Effective method of intervention (vaccination); elimination has been achieved in some countries in the Caribbean and the Americas as a result of immunization.

Measles shares these features with smallpox, which has been eradicted globally, but, as predicted, measles eradication is proving more difficult — partly because it is much more infectious than smallpox and partly because there is a window of vulnerability between the duration of protection by maternal antibody (and concomitant resistance to measles vaccination) and attainment of the age of 12 months, at which time vaccination is assured of being effective. Because of the inevitability of repeated reintroduction of infection, countrywide elimination does not constitute a satisfactory outcome, except as a preliminary step to global eradication. Some innovative measures for improving vaccine coverage capitalize on strategies developed during the poliomyelitis eradication campaign. In addition to its intrinsic importance, a campaign to eradicate measles by mass vaccination with a combined vaccine may simplify the eradication of rubella and, potentially, mumps as well.

Rubella

Although not listed as the second candidate, I will consider rubella next, because the campaign to eradicate it could usefully be linked with the measles eradication programme. Rubella resembles measles not only in having a generalized rash, but also in being a specifically human, acute, self-limiting disease, except that the rare cases of congenital infection may continue to excrete virus for years. Although it is suspected to be a potential trigger for autoimmune diseases, acute rubella is a trivial disease, hardly worth worrying about; however, congenital rubella is a severe disease. Since postnatal rubella is such a mild disease, with many subclinical cases, effective surveillance will be difficult. It might be useful to link the countrywide elimination and ultimate global eradication of rubella with that of

[1] Visiting Fellow, John Curtin School of Medical Research, Australian National University, Canberra, Australia.

measles, by using a combined measles–rubella vaccine, or even better, a measles–rubella–mumps vaccine, so as to minimize the numbers of inoculations. It may be that this scheme is not practicable or too costly, but the chance of eliminating and subsequently eradicating three diseases "at the cost of one" makes the use of a triple vaccine attractive. Since measles is probably the most highly infectious of these three diseases, and the most easily recognized, a good surveillance system for measles might prove to be an effective surrogate for good surveillance for rubella and mumps as well as in judging the efficacy of immunization campaigns.

The eradication of rubella, like measles, calls for an intensive, relatively short campaign, so that all countries can maintain their enthusiasm and commitment.

Hepatitis B

Like measles and smallpox, hepatitis B virus is a specifically human pathogen and a good vaccine is available. It is clearly a major disease burden in countries where it is common. However, unlike any of the other viral diseases cited by the survey teams, it is a disease in which many persons, especially those infected in infancy, become chronically infected and are persistent or recurrent excretors of the virus. This presents a particularly difficult problem for surveillance, requiring careful laboratory screening on large numbers of infants and older people, most of whom are not sick. Inclusion of hepatitis B vaccination in the EPI schedule, as proposed by WHO, would be a valuable first step towards control. However, many countries in which the incidence is low are reluctant to spend the money needed for vaccination against a disease that does not present them with a substantial health problem; yet, if eradication is to be achieved, an early start in all countries is highly desirable.

Countrywide elimination of hepatitis B requires countries to enter into programmes that call for a long-term commitment, over decades, to outlast cases of chronic infection already present in the population at the start of the programme. This is something that will be difficult to ensure even in the absence of war or serious civil disturbances, which experience in the last 50 years suggests are inevitable. Nevertheless, there is every reason to encourage more countries to include hepatitis B vaccine in their childhood immunization schedules, as suggested by WHO. Countries where the disease is common should be encouraged to screen for chronic hepatitis B infection in pregnant women and vaccinate their infants at birth.

Yellow fever

In 1801 Jenner made the optimistic statement: "it now becomes too manifest to admit of controversy, that the annihilation of the Small Pox, the most dreadful scourge of the human species, must be the final result of this practice" (vaccination). A hundred and seventy-six years later, his prediction was realized. The next disease for which such a forecast was made was yellow fever (3). After eliminating yellow fever from Havana and controlling it in Panama, Gorgas wrote in his report in July 1902: "I look forward in the future to a time when yellow fever will have entirely disappeared as a disease to which mankind is subject." After a visit to Asia in 1914, Dr W. Rose, Director of the International Health Commission of the newly established Rockefeller Foundation, found that health officials there were profoundly concerned that yellow fever might be brought to Asia as a consequence of the opening of the Panama Canal that year and the resulting increase in maritime traffic. After consultation with Gorgas, by now Surgeon-General of the United States Army, Rose promised the Rockefeller Foundation's help in the global eradication of yellow fever. This prospect was based on control of the urban mosquito *Aedes aegypti*, which was thought to be the only vector. It was believed that there were a few endemic centres of disease that served as seedbeds, and that if they were destroyed, yellow fever would disappear forever. Early efforts in South America were dramatically successful, but then there were disturbing small outbreaks in forest areas, where *A. aegypti* could not be found. Although this situation had been first reported in Colombia in 1907, it was not until 1932 that Soper obtained definitive evidence that monkeys constituted a jungle reservoir of yellow fever, and all hopes of global eradication of the disease were dispelled.

This piece of history is relevant for two reasons. First, although the fact sheet prepared for this conference speaks of elimination rather than eradication, if we follow the definitions of the Dahlem Workshop, "control" would be a better term than elimination. Second, I believe that in addition to preventing unnecessary illness and death in Africa and South America, a major reason for pressing ahead with efforts at controlling the disease (this time by vaccination rather than mosquito control) is to prevent its spread to Asia. Rose was concerned about this in 1914; I participated in a conference in Kuala Lumpur in 1954 to discuss the same problem, and here we are again discussing it in 1998. It would be disastrous to see the spread of yellow fever in the reverse direction to that of dengue and dengue haemorrhagic fever over the last 20 years. This is an additional reason for trying to improve the coverage of vaccination in Africa and South America.

In 1988, WHO and UNICEF recommended routine childhood and catch-up yellow fever vaccination in Africa, but coverage rates are still low. Although the 17D vaccine is probably the best live virus vaccine that has ever been developed, there may be problems in using it in infants and immunosuppressed persons (4). This matter should be investigated, and if there is a significant risk, the potential of a recombinant vaccine or a DNA vaccine should be considered.

General comments

Smallpox was successfully eradicated because it was a specifically human disease, with no subclinical cases so that effective surveillance was relatively easy, there was a good vaccine with production facilities in many countries, and the wealthy countries had a strong self-interest in supporting eradication — to free them from the necessity of vaccinating outgoing travellers and the danger of importations. Poliomyelitis is proving more difficult than smallpox (5), because there are so many subclinical infections, but has the great advantage that there is an excellent oral vaccine.

Because there is an animal reservoir for yellow fever virus, only three of the four viral diseases listed for discussion could be "eradicated." For all four, there is an effective method of intervention, namely a good vaccine, although improvements could be made. Each of the three eradicable diseases presents problems. For measles, the main problem is to ensure the political and financial support required to achieve and maintain high immunization levels in both industrialized and developing countries, which are necessary because of its extremely high infectivity. As with all specifically human infectious diseases, the desirability of targeting eradication rather than countrywide elimination is underlined by the frequent reports of measles outbreaks in countries with low levels of the diseases, due to the arrival by air from other countries of infected persons during the incubation period.

For rubella, the difficulty of diagnosis, and hence of surveillance, constitute the principal problem. An eradication programme might be more effective if, instead of having to mount a rather difficult surveillance programme for rubella, the campaign was linked with the measles eradication campaign by the use of a combined vaccine, a measles–rubella or a measles–mumps–rubella vaccine. For hepatitis B, the prolonged infectivity of chronic cases constitutes a problem in that it calls for a very long-term commitment for continued universal childhood vaccination, as well as vaccination at birth of infants born by mothers who are carriers of hepatitis B virus.

However, by far the most important difficulty with all elimination/eradication programmes is the cost, which is beyond the resources of the poor countries. None of these diseases presents the risk to the wealthy countries that smallpox did, hence it is proving much more difficult to persuade these countries to expand their moral and financial support to the extent that will be required for the eradication of measles, let alone hepatitis B and rubella. The political will is lacking. Despite the cost, it would to be highly desirable to tie efforts to eliminate and ultimately eradicate as many diseases as possible together, by using combination vaccines such as measles–mumps–rubella.

Control of yellow fever appears to be a more practicable proposition, but judging by the response to the 1988 recommendation of WHO/UNICEF, the countries most concerned do not appear to be seized of its value. They need support not only from the wealthy countries, but also, on grounds of self-interest, from the countries most at risk of its extension, namely countries in Asia whose territories include areas infested with *A. aegypti*.

References

1. **Dowdle WR, Hopkins DR.** eds. *The eradication of infectious diseases: report of the Dahlem Workshop on the Eradication of Infectious Diseases*. Chichester, John Wiley & Sons, 1998.
2. **de Quadros CA et al.** Measles eradication: experience in the Americas. In: Global Disease Elimination and Eradication as Public Health Strategies. *Bulletin of the World Health Organization*, 1998, **76** (Suppl. 2): 47–52.
3. **Strode GK.** ed. *Yellow fever*. New York, McGraw-Hill, 1951.
4. **Tsai TF.** Yellow fever (fact sheet). In: Global Disease Elimination and Eradication as Public Health Strategies. *Bulletin of the World Health Organization*, 1998, **76** (Suppl. 2): 158–159.
5. **Hull HF et al.** Perspectives from the global poliomyelitis eradication initiative. In: Global Disease Elimination and Eradication as Public Health Strategies. *Bulletin of the World Health Organization*, 1998, **76** (Suppl. 2): 42–46.

REPORTS OF THE WORKGROUPS

Report of the Workgroup on Disease Elimination/ Eradication and Sustainable Health Development

D. Salisbury[1]

Introduction

Eradication initiatives have been both applauded for their successes (smallpox, poliomyelitis) and criticized for their failings (malaria, smallpox). The Workgroup on Disease Elimination/Eradication and Sustainable Health Development tried to identify the critical components of policy development, human resource utilization, financing and sustainability that contribute to prospects for success. Subgroups worked on each of the topics against a set of core questions (see Table 1).

Policy and strategy

General principles

Disease eradication is distinct from disease control. Terms such as "elimination" or "elimination as a public health problem" are often confusing and are best understood as subcategories of disease control. Their use should be avoided as far as possible, which leaves only eradication initiatives and ongoing disease control programmes as alternatives.

Because eradication programmes differ, it is difficult to generalize about them. Some diseases for eradication are of global importance, while others may be of regional or local importance. How much emphasis is accorded to health system strengthening as an objective of eradication may vary depending on this fact and other features described by other work groups.

Eradication programmes cannot correct the deficiencies of existing health systems. Their objectives should be: 1) reduction of the target disease to zero incidence, and maintaining this when all interventions have ceased; and 2) strengthening and further development of health systems so that other disease control programmes and health system functions (e.g. monitoring and surveillance, supervision, and programme management) will also benefit from the eradication effort.

Themes

The group agreed that eradication programmes, besides reducing the incidence of a target disease to zero even after the discontinuation of control measures, have the potential to contribute greatly to the strengthening of health systems. These potential benefits should be identified and delineated at the start of any eradication initiative. As must be done for the disease eradication objective, measurable targets for achieving these development benefits should be set and the programme should be held accountable for their realization.

Recommendations

• Eradication initiatives should be implemented with the support of a broad coalition of partners. Great efforts should be made to build consensus and a shared sense of mission among United Nations agencies, the donor community (both public and private sector), and participating countries.

• Managers of eradication initiatives should respect the importance of other, ongoing public health programmes being promoted and implemented by the ministry of health and by other staff, internationally, nationally, and locally.

• To the extent possible, peripheral level decision-makers should be allowed to reach centrally established targets in a flexible and locally appropriate way. Similarly, when centrally driven priorities are set, those with responsibility at the peripheral level, who may have considerable autonomy for resource allocation, should understand their role within the wider objective.

• Successful eradication programmes are good examples of effective management. The programme activities should further the development of leadership and managerial skills among health personnel, building programme management capacities which the staff involved can carry to other health programmes.

• Surveillance of programmatic processes and outcomes (reduced morbidity and mortality) is important for successful eradication. The initiatives must demonstrate the principles of effective surveillance and actively develop and implement surveillance sys-

---

[1] Principal Medical Officer, Department of Health, London, England.

Table 1: **Disease eradication and sustainable health development**

Subgroup concentrations
- Overall health policy (international, national and local):   Group A
  strategic planning, organization of systems, management
  processes
- Finance and resource mobilization   Group B
- Human resources: training and social mobilization   Group C
- Health services: provision, management, and performance   Group D

Core questions
- What does eradication strengthen?
- What does eradication risk?
- What synergies can be developed in eradication activities?
- Will the shift from public sector service provision for primary care and maternal and child health be significant for eradication activities?
- Given decentralization of responsibilities for public health, how will the momentum be achieved for eradication activities, when the central public health role has diminished?
- When responsibilities for resource allocation are delivered at the local level, in line with local health needs, how will global eradication priorities be "imposed" when they are not perceived as locally important?
- Will the greatest challenges to eradication activities come from those whose services are least well developed?
  - Will industrialized countries compromise eradication activities because they do not perceive the need to divert resources to diseases of little consequence to themselves?
  - How will they be influenced to accept the real and opportunity costs when they see little direct personal benefit?
  - How can commitment be assured in advance of establishing eradication goals?
  - Can we identify a set of prerequisites or preconditions that must be satisfied, before a new eradication goal is set? Is this worthwhile?
  - How can we ensure that quality is improved by the achievement of eradication?
  - Are there essential requirements that should already be in place before eradication activities begin?
  - What might such indicators be?
  - How can we encourage those for whom eradication activities might be the most difficult to be in the forefront? Should they be?
  - Can we make specific recommendations that will ensure that health care systems achieve the maximum benefits from eradication activities?

tems which can readily be adapted to meet the needs of other national priority programmes after eradication is achieved.

Tensions

An eradication programme has the potential to produce substantial benefits to a health system beyond its disease-specific goals, but the following tensions are inherent to any consideration of whether to undertake an eradication initiative.

- Since other programmes will inevitably be sacrificed or delayed when an eradication goal is pursued, these opportunity costs should carefully be analysed prior to embarking upon an eradication initiative.

- The desire to show initial successes by starting an eradication initiative in the better prepared countries is balanced by the fact that less developed countries need more time to realize fully the potential benefits of eradication. Yet frequently, as is the case with poliomyelitis eradication, the countries which need the most time to develop sustainable surveillance systems, to raise vaccination coverage levels through routine vaccination programmes, and to strengthen programme management are paradoxically those which are accorded the least amount of

time in which to attain disease eradication goals. Strategies, including flexibility in timing the introduction of interventions in order to achieve reductions in disease incidence and to strengthen the health system, should be developed to ensure that all countries benefit from participation in the programme.

- A balance must be achieved between two contrasting positions. First, some persons advocate eradication only when two outcomes can be assured, namely the absence of disease and the attainment of specific health service gains identified in advance of commencement of the eradication effort. Second, there is the view of the primacy of the eradication goal with a subsidiary objective of expected health service gains, which cannot be measured before the intervention commences. This exemplifies the tensions inherent in considering eradication targets.

Health systems and support

Assessment

Planners must assess the capacity of the current system to meet the requirements of the eradication intervention and identify opportunities for capacity building. Within existing systems, different levels of capacity exist in various countries. Planners need to assess objectively the operational levels of the system relative to the eradication objectives. This will include personnel available, cold chain integrity (if required), costs of delivery, transport requirements, other logistic needs, seasonal variations in epidemiology and transmission, anticipated opportunity costs, and social factors which may facilitate or impede achievement of the programme's objectives.

Once the assessment is complete, decision-makers must weigh the pros and cons of the eradication platform and decide whether to proceed or invest in pre-eradication interventions which will strengthen the system and enable a more effective and efficient eradication effort.

Time frame

A time frame must be developed to sequence rationally the events towards eradication, and to improve the standards of delivery (e.g. logistics and supply, high quality service delivery, injection safety) and maximize the use of appropriate technologies. Planners must consider the sequence of events to implement the eradication programme relative to the operational requirements of the intervention. Cofactors within the eradication's operational structure should also be emphasized and applied within the existing health system to improve delivery standards. Appropriate technologies (e.g. VVMs, single-use syringes, drug inventory systems) should be considered and highlighted, as appropriate, to maximize delivery and improve the efficiency of eradication efforts and routine services.

Planning and design

Planning and design must maximize the partnerships of all potential stakeholders including the community, schoolchildren, local government, NGOs, and the private sector. Partnership is the key to effective eradication and control programmes. For the eradication programme, planners, decision-makers and donors must identify suitable partnerships among private and public sector colleagues. The essence of workable partnerships must include a common, long-term commitment to the eradication platform, clear lines of responsibility among partners (based on respective comparative advantages), and, on-the-ground planning of interventions.

Clear agreement on impact indicators, benchmarks of progress, key results, and the performance of each partner will favour smooth implementation

and enable discrete and empirical assessments of each partner's input and output. Working together to achieve a common goal is a strong advantage of eradication programmes; coupled to system strengthening, this becomes a powerful combination to achieve sustainable success within a reasonable time frame. Clear examples should be drawn from the poliomyelitis eradication experience to enunciate the nature of workable partnerships and an empirical appraisal of sustainable, system-strengthening impact.

Quality of delivery

For eradication, the quality of delivery (safety, coverage, effectiveness and efficiency) must be ensured. Quality assurance is a key aspect of eradication and control programmes. The eradication effort must first assess the quality, stability, financing and efficiency of national programmes, and identify any weak points.

If safety issues arise, either from injections or drug distribution, planners and donors must proceed with caution or postpone embarking on the eradication effort until a reasonable level of confidence is displayed by all partners. Efforts must not be jeopardized by uncertainties related to quality, delivery, assessment and/or impact. Embarking prematurely, without proper consideration of quality, safety, effectiveness and efficiency, can result in extended efforts with higher costs, less system strengthening, and poor planning and judgement. Positive lessons from the poliomyelitis eradication initiative should be identified and applied to ensure future quality, safety, effectiveness and efficiency.

Monitoring systems

Eradication requires the development of monitoring systems that use quantitative and qualitative indicators to identify gaps between standards and performance. These data must be used to improve and sustain the quality of delivery systems in a continuing process. Monitoring systems must be put in place to track the approved indicators of both performance and impact. Without quantitative indicators that focus on quality, the benefits of the eradication effort will be compromised. Although eradication need not solve the problems of health systems, it must ensure the quality of delivery, and impart a lasting impact in terms of human, logistic, administrative, and technical processes. From the initial planning phases, empirical benchmarks of quality must be derived and monitored.

Surveillance

Any eradication programme must include "surveillance for action" both for the eradication and for the development of the surveillance infrastructure, which includes all stakeholders (i.e. public and private). For example, detection of a case of acute flaccid paralysis needs to include a response at each level of the system — that is, parental instructions at the household level, investigation, laboratory collection, reporting at the district level, and appropriate mop-up. "Surveillance for action" thus encompasses system strengthening, information flow, and response. The positive development and impact of a grass-roots surveillance system is clear. Every effort should be made among partners to establish a sensitive and specific surveillance system that responds to unusual events.

Investments that promote sustainability through self-reliance, must be pursued in contrast to top-down, donor-driven efforts that impart little lasting impact. Lessons must be gleaned from the Latin American experience to ensure that appropriately strengthened surveillance systems are put in place which can serve routine systems elsewhere and future eradication efforts in general. Every effort should be made to document the success and short-comings of the poliomyelitis eradication initiative regarding surveillance and certification.

Applied research

Eradication must support applied research in the field to identify strategies, and track the effectiveness and efficiency of delivery of the interventions. Applied and operations research must be conducted to improve the effectiveness of administrative and technical interventions. This research must be oriented towards practical issues which will drive the eradication effort forwards and improve technical, operational, and fiscal efficiencies. Data must provide an empirical basis for decision-making, particularly when assessing the cost and cost-benefits of specific programmes.

Much applied research should be conducted prior to the launch of the eradication effort to ensure the accuracy of the approach and provide baseline information that can be used in monitoring the impact. Once efforts are under way, prospective research agenda should be developed to track impact, identify efficiency paradigms, and strengthen delivery. This research should serve to improve system quality, while fine tuning eradication interventions.

Financing and resource mobilization

Benefits and dangers

What does eradication bring to health programme financing?

• Additional mobilization of resources (both financial and human) at global, national and local levels, from public and private sources, for both additional (eradication-related) costs and basic service costs.

• Additional partnerships, including those committed to resource mobilization, leading to significantly greater numbers of volunteers and other people involved in health action.

• Attention to sponsorship and other innovative financing mechanisms.

• The capacities to identify progress and sustain donor interest in health financing.

• Clear end-points and time frames that minimize discussions of sustainability.

• Increased public visibility and support for health, including increased willingness to pay for health services, as well as increased international solidarity with global health issues.

What are the actual and potential dangers of eradication for the health system and health development?

• Diversion of resources (financial/human) from existing support to basic services nationally and internationally, and overall reduced attention to meeting the resource needs of basic services. Each activity that is employed in furtherance of an eradication objective may reflect an opportunity cost. These opportunity costs are significant in all health service systems, from the most sophisticated, where high levels of disease control may exist, to emerging health care systems that may be quite vulnerable to the diversion of scarce skills.

• Opportunities "foregone", especially in countries where the eradication effort has a low impact in terms of health outcomes.

• Potential decreases in resources available for research, both for the eradication effort and for other health problems.

• Failure to estimate accurately the needs of the eradication efforts, leading to subsequent "forced" diversions once effort is underway.

• Enthusiasm for eradication could lead to many simultaneous eradication efforts and induce failure.

Recommendations

Based on the above points, the following recommendations aim at maximizing benefits and minimizing dangers.

• Early planning for eradication and basic health services to accurately identify the costs and benefits. In particular, planning should include: long-term costs for strengthening the health system and additional costs for the eradication effort; evaluation of current budgets and capacities (national and international); financial and human resource needs; individual and societal benefits; cost-effectiveness and affordability of the proposed eradication effort; and specific cost criteria for evaluating the performance of the eradication effort (e.g. cost per child protected in various situations, by country).

• Articulation of the rationale and criteria for provision of external support for eradication efforts, which are not affordable from national sources, and mobilization of external resources, including the cost and benefit of eradication to industrialized countries. Many industrialized countries contribute significantly to resource mobilization for eradication activities; however, within some countries there may be considerable resistance to diverting resources from health service activities when initiating eradication efforts if the disease burden is perceived to be low and the opportunity cost of the attainment of eradication is perceived to be high.

• Early recruitment of partners, especially in the private sector, and identification of innovative financing mechanisms.

• Ongoing advocacy based on successes, to recruit new partners and resources, and assessment of public attitudes towards funding in both developing and industrialized countries.

• Mechanisms for ongoing and periodic financial review and resource coordination, review and updating of cost criteria.

• Ways of maintaining, within the health sector, any resource savings gained from eradication efforts (this rarely occurs since real term costs for eradication frequently fall to health ministries, while the health gains accrue to national treasuries or ministries of trade). Furthermore, increased public awareness as a consequence of eradication activities may lead to increased willingness to provide resources for basic services.

• Global, regional, and local resource mobilization reviews should be planned.

• Resources for eradication activities should be additional to those available for basic health care services and should not be provided at the detriment of existing services or those that are planned.

• A careful, transparent process for decision-making on new eradication efforts, based inter alia on the following: assessment of the global capacities for resources mobilization and financing; assessment of opportunity costs, at national and global levels; opportunities for public health synergy of different eradication efforts; and the need to balance the requirements of centrally driven goals with the potentially very different peripheral level priorities.

Human resource development, training, and community mobilization

Themes

The Workgroup considered that eradication programmes have great potential to strengthen the capacity of health services by training health workers, recruiting community members for health improvement, and providing concrete examples of good management. It is often assumed that eradication programmes will improve human resources. While this sometimes happens, it would be more efficient to include capacity building in the design of eradication programmes. This would increase the probability that these desirable benefits are, in fact, achieved.

Explicit planning for capacity building will focus the attention of planners on potential negative features of eradication programmes, which could be avoided. While it is unreasonable to burden eradication programmes with improving the primary health care (PHC) package, these programmes should contribute to the maintenance and strengthening of health service structures.

Human resource development

Eradication programmes often create a brain drain by diverting talent and human resources away from PHC programmes. In response to these problems, the recommendations outlined below were suggested.

• Incentive systems that encourage and reward personnel to seek out and capitalize on opportunities for synergy and integration of health services with eradication programmes should be developed.

• Supervisory systems need to be able to reward integration.

• Eradication programmes must invest in building basic human infrastructure. There should be clear human development objectives in all programmes which should be evaluated to meeting human resource needs. Any new eradication effort must train and develop the human resource pool as part of the initial stages of capacity building for delivering the basic package of health services (e.g. HIS, logistics, training, and evaluation).

• Eradication programmes should not attempt to build temporary or parallel structures whereby human resources are fostered and then jettisoned.

• The district and community levels have a critical role in sustainability of services and successful implementation of eradication objectives. While the central level is also important, human resource development and training need to focus on those at district and community levels.

• If eradication campaigns need to be sustained and external support is not available, it is essential that they be integrated with local health provision capacity.

Training

Eradication programmes tend to retain a hierarchical division of labour, with assessment and planning/policy skills at the national level and implementation of skills at the district or local level. Most developing countries are undergoing decentralization and are rapidly shifting responsibilities to the periphery for planning/policy development, problem solving, and health problem assessment; the present training infrastructure is addressing this growing need. Training curricula and infrastructure should be modified to reflect these changing roles and responsibilities. These include new skills at the local level which must take advantage of emerging technologies (e.g. the Internet, distance-based learning) to reach large numbers with standardized curricula. Eradication programmes tend to create parallel (and even redundant) training curricula and infrastructure which may be wasteful and not sustainable, and which work against the integration of functions. Based on these considerations, the following recommendations were made.

• Training in areas such as management (including that of quality assurance), leadership, and epidemiology should be generic and offered in integrated courses to employees from different health service backgrounds; this training should focus on the practical skills needed by workers to do their jobs. Indicators of the outcome of training should be linked to the programme's goals (i.e. programme achievements reflect training attainments).

• Training for eradication programmes should provide skills that can be used in implementing other programmes.

• Training programmes should have specific objectives in terms of impact, increases in programme output and competencies. Evaluation should be based on the accomplishment of these goals.

• Training should include skills for social mobilization, health outreach, health education, and health promotion.

• Training needs to have a practical component so that trainees bring real skills, not just theoretical knowledge to the job.

• Training must be appropriate for each level and should seek to minimize the boundary between community volunteers and beginners among health workers.

• Practical experience should be an important criterion for entrance into the health workforce and practical competencies should be a major criterion for evaluation.

• Training should be problem-oriented and focused on knowledge and competencies for improving health in the specific programme, but which can also be applied to other health programmes.

• Training should be designed and evaluated with clear objectives in terms of competencies and expected outputs.

• Training should include not only specific technical information, but also competencies in problem-solving, decision-making, and management in the health system. Training should include descriptions of the competencies required and constraints of the management level directly above the trainees.

Community mobilization

Since eradication programmes may mobilize communities for eradication goals without building community support and capacity for other health goals, the points shown below should be taken into account.

• Social mobilization should emphasize that people are being mobilized for improved health, not just for a specific programme. Use of non-health personnel has long-term benefits in terms of sustainability and community support.

• Training that furthers the skills of social mobilization should incorporate wider competencies than those simply required for the eradication objective, and should be general rather than specific so that they can be used in the future for sustainability of health services after the eradication objective has been achieved.

• Health education should reflect community concerns.

• Eradication programmes should express their goals in terms the community can understand.

• The successes of health care workers and volunteers should be documented and given recognition.

Conclusions

Overall

There are intrinsic and unavoidable tensions between the concepts of eradication and sustainable health development. These tensions arise because of polarization between vertical and integrated approaches — specific rather than comprehensive goals, "top-down" rather than "bottom-up" directions, and a time-limited rather than long-term agenda. It is essential to acknowledge and overcome these tensions so that eradication programmes can contribute to health development. In addition, the following beliefs and acts of faith accompany eradication programmes: first, there is a legacy of wider benefits than simply the achievement of eradication or complete absence of cases; second, the cost–benefit of eradication is greater compared with the achievement of high levels of control; and third, commitment must be made on the grounds of beliefs or, alternatively, further eradication endeavours must be postponed until the prerequisites can be confirmed.

Besides gaining insight into the technical feasibility of eradication, rules are being developed that create a discipline that was not previously acknowledged. These rules encompass resource mobilization, strategic planning, human resources and training, and social mobilization. Detailed, meticulous planning is essential to take full advantage of the opportunities created by eradication programmes, thereby avoiding the potential for unwanted, negative effects. However, the experience with eradication programmes to date has shown some of the limitations of the planning process.

Ideally, the potential benefits of eradication to health development should be identified at the outset. Similar to the eradication targets, measurable targets should be set for achieving these benefits. The eradication programme should be held accountable for the attainment of these wider objectives. Resources for eradication activities should be additional to those available for basic health care services

and should in no way be detrimental to existing services or those that are planned, except in situations where the consequences have been carefully considered.

Health policy/health systems

• Eradication programmes should not be held responsible for curing the ills of existing health systems.

• Eradication programmes should have two objectives: 1) reduction of the target disease to zero incidence, which can be maintained even when all intervention ceases; and 2) further development and strengthening of health systems, especially with regard to monitoring and surveillance, supervision, and programme management.

• Eradication initiatives should be implemented with the support of a broad coalition of partners; great efforts should be made to build consensus.

• Managers of eradication initiatives should respect the importance of other, ongoing public health programmes.

• To the extent possible, peripheral-level decision-makers should be allowed to reach centrally established targets in a flexible and locally appropriate way.

• Successful eradication programmes are powerful examples of effective management, building management capacities to be carried to other health programmes.

• Efforts should be made to design eradication programme activities that further the development of leadership and managerial and technical skills among health personnel.

• Eradication initiatives should actively participate in the development and implementation of effective surveillance systems which can be readily adapted to meet the needs of other national priority programmes after eradication is achieved.

Human resources, training and social mobilization

It is essential for eradication programmes to include the following features.

• Training in management, quality assurance, leadership and epidemiology should be generally available and offered in integrated courses.

• Training for eradication programmes should explicitly cover skills that can be widely used;

acquired knowledge and competencies have to apply to other health programmes as well.

• Social mobilization has to be for improved health, and not only for a specific programme, involving non-health personnel, because of long-term benefits in terms of sustainability, community support, and epidemiological surveillance.

It is essential for eradication programmes to avoid the following pitfalls.

• Capacity building without appropriate attention to health information systems and evaluation.

• Building parallel or temporary structures whereby human resources are fostered and jettisoned.

• Concentrating on the central level and over-looking the need to remember human resources at district and community levels.

Financing and resource mobilization

The benefits eradication brings to health programme financing include those outlined below.

• Additional resource mobilization at global, national, and local levels for both further eradication and basic service costs.

• Innovative financing mechanisms (e.g. sponsorship).

• The capacities to identify progress and sustain donor interest in health financing.

Actual and potential dangers of eradication for the health system and health development include those mentioned below.

• Opportunities "foregone", especially for countries in which the eradication effort has a low impact in terms of health outcomes.

• Failure to accurately estimate the needs of the eradication efforts, leading to subsequent "forced" resource diversions once the effort is underway.

Planning

Early planning is needed to identify accurately costs (both long-term for strengthening the health system and additional costs for the eradication effort) and benefits. Planning should include the following.

• Evaluation of current budgets and capacities (national and international).

• Financial and human resource needs.

• Cost-effectiveness and affordability of the proposed eradication effort.

• Specific cost criteria for evaluation of performance of the eradication effort (e.g. the cost of a child protected for various country situations).

• A careful, transparent process for decision-making on new eradication efforts, based *inter alia* on factors such as assessment of the global capacities for resource mobilization and financing; assessment of opportunity costs at national and global levels; opportunities for public health synergy of different eradication efforts; and the need to balance the requirements of centrally driven goals with the potentially very different peripheral level priorities — especially important when decentralization leads to district level autonomy in resource prioritization.

Development of sustainable health services

• Planners must assess the capacity of the current system to meet the requirements of the eradication intervention and identify opportunities for capacity building.

• Planning and design must maximize the partnerships of all potential stakeholders.

• Eradication must ensure the quality of delivery regarding safety, coverage, effectiveness, and efficiency.

• Any eradication programme must include "surveillance for action" — both for eradication and for development of the surveillance infrastructure including all public and private sector stakeholders.

• Countries must carefully weigh the consequences of their eventual decision to adhere to an eradication initiative, and consider the value of strengthening their health systems as a contribution to the success of the eradication programme. Similarly, eradication initiatives can contribute to strengthening health services and these benefits should be identified whenever possible.

• Eradication should remain exceptional and be carefully designed to maximize the chances of success and positive effects for sustainable health development.

Acknowledgements

I should like to thank Dr Denis Broun (Chairman), Dr Victor Barbiero, Dr Ron Waldman, Dr Mark White, and Dr Roy Widdus for their special contributions to this report.

Report of the Workgroup on Noninfectious Diseases

M.M. Dayrit[1]

Introduction

The Workgroup on Noninfectious Diseases recognized that the strategies for eradication and elimination of infectious diseases would need to be revised when applied to noninfectious diseases. The group divided itself into four subgroups to discuss the following: 1) a conceptual framework for eradication/elimination strategies as applied to noninfectious diseases, 2) toxic exposures, 3) protein–energy malnutrition, and 4) micronutrient malnutrition.

The group noted that the definition for "eradication" from the Dahlem Workshop — "zero cases, zero risk, cessation of intervention" — would not apply to noninfectious diseases. The conditions considered for eradication so far have been diseases or "portions of diseases" that have a single cause (e.g. cases of acute flaccid paralysis caused by poliovirus). Some noninfectious diseases (e.g. certain toxic exposures) may qualify for eradication because they have a single cause which could be removed completely (e.g. 2-naphthylamine-induced cancer). However, most noninfectious diseases (e.g. resulting from nutritional deficiency) cannot be "eradicated" because the intervention measures must be continued to ensure that the deficiencies do not recur.

The group recognized that there would be difficulty in the strict application to noninfectious diseases of the term "elimination", defined as "zero cases, continuing risk, continuing intervention". For example, micronutrient supplementation, when given to a population with different levels of nutritional adequacy, may not help those with severe deficiency. Furthermore, fluctuations in the adequacy of the diet and supplementation could lead to a rise in cases periodically. However, the group felt that the use of "elimination", despite the technical definition, in relation to nutritional deficiencies and other noninfectious diseases deserved some consideration because of its value as a communications and political tool for rallying enthusiasm, resources and support.

Because noninfectious diseases do not fit the strict definition for candidate diseases to be eradi-

cated or eliminated, the group agreed that other criteria were necessary in setting priorities and in competing for resources. These criteria include burden of disease, cost-effectiveness of interventions, political commitment, and social acceptability which, the group emphasized, had to be considered regardless of whether a disease could be eradicated or eliminated.

Facilitating and mitigating factors

The Workgroup considered that one important factor affecting the success of disease control efforts is the degree of interdependence among communities in terms of community interventions. This interdependence appeared to be less for noninfectious than for infectious diseases. For example, the failure of one community to control nutritional deficiencies in its population did not necessarily result in a negative impact on the incidence of disease in a neighbouring community. In contrast, failure of poliomyelitis eradication in one country may pose a continuing risk to its neighbours. For occupational and environmental diseases, exposures in one community may affect health in another community (e.g. a worker taking home a toxin on his contaminated clothing, or a toxin from a factory affecting distant, downwind communities). In comparison to infectious diseases, the relative lack of international interdependence concerning noninfectious diseases may provide greater latitude for one country to select its own health priorities unfettered by the health situation of others. However, the lower degree of interdependence among communities might result in weaker external support.

Another factor affecting the implementation of programmes for noninfectious diseases, which was emphasized, is that the resources from the health system budget to sustain interventions for some noncommunicable diseases (e.g. micronutrient deficiencies) may be reduced after resources from other sectors are tapped. For example, once the private sector has begun iodizing salt and the distribution systems are in place to make it universally available in a country, the need for iodine supplementation campaigns would diminish. Furthermore, given that a nutritional intervention (e.g. salt iodization) is safe,

[1] Vice President, Medical Services Division, Aetna Health Care, Inc., Makati City, Philippines.

effective and generally applicable, and also that the disease (e.g. iodine deficiency) is noncommunicable, highly sensitive and specific surveillance systems would be less critical than would be the case for the elimination or eradication of a communicable infectious disease.

The group concluded that three issues are critical when considering eradication and elimination strategies for noninfectious diseases: 1) the enormous diversity of these diseases — each one must be evaluated according to its own characteristics; 2) national health priorities — these have to be evaluated and interventions need community acceptance within the cultural context of each country; and 3) the need for interventions for proven effectiveness — countries and donors will be unlikely to invest in interventions that cannot be shown to be effective.

Toxic exposures

The subgroup recognized the long tradition of successful international efforts to control specific occupational and environmental exposures and national efforts to control other exposure hazards. Examples of international elimination of exposure include phosphorus in the manufacture of matches, and certain synthetic organic dyes that cause bladder cancer; successful national efforts have eliminated silicosis among workers engaged in sandblasting.

As the number of potential toxic-agent candidates for elimination is large and the selection of candidate exposures is difficult, three general points were considered. First, because of uncertainty in the extent of exposure to toxic agents, the number of individuals exposed worldwide to selected occupational and environmental toxins had to be properly estimated. Second, correct estimates had to be made about the number of incident and prevalent cases. Third, exposures resulting in high rates of diseases, albeit in relatively small populations (e.g. certain synthetic specialty chemicals), were considered to qualify as candidates, as well as other toxins that affect large numbers of people (e.g. silica and asbestos).

The occupational and environmental exposures that were considered varied in the magnitude of related cases, evidence of preventability either at particular worksites or countrywide, and the reliability of the known exposure and morbidity statistics about each condition. Considering all these factors, the group recommended two initial candidates for global elimination: lead poisoning and silicosis, because of their seriousness, the existence of a substan-

tial fund of knowledge about these exposures, and the demonstration of control at national level, in the case of silicosis, resulting from a previous WHO commitment to this problem.

Lead poisoning

Lead poisoning affects both children and workers. An impressive body of data exists on the adverse health effects of lead poisoning, especially in children, even at very low levels of exposure (as low as $10\,\mu g/dl$). The negative impact of lead exposure on the cognitive development of children argues for the integration of lead poisoning prevention with comprehensive programmes to prevent mental impairment (e.g. prevention of iodine deficiency and iron deficiency). This argument is further enhanced by the fact that adequate levels of iron and calcium reduce lead uptake in the gut.

Various interventions have effectively reduced or eliminated lead poisoning from paint and additives in fuel, exposure from radiator and battery repairs, etc. Several countries have effectively controlled, if not eliminated, occupational and environmental lead poisoning. Models for lead poisoning prevention exist in the successful programmes in the USA and certain northern European countries (principally Scandinavia), which have reduced blood lead levels in the general population, especially young children, and in occupationally exposed adults.

Techniques for the determination of lead in blood and in the environment are well established in the developed world, but need to be established globally along with quality assurance networks. Recent availability of rugged, low-cost, easy-to-operate lead measurement devices make assessment of human lead exposure feasible in a variety of settings. Effective treatments (succimer and EDTA) are available for children with elevated blood lead levels.

The strategies outlined below were recommended.

- *Assessment* through targeted and nationally representative sample surveys to determine the extent of the problem in countries.

- *Analysis* of data to refine targets for intervention and determine the most susceptible populations in a given area.

- *Action* to eliminate lead from gasoline, paint, water sources and pipes, food cans, and industrial sources through legislation, regulation and education; to abate existing sources of lead in the environment (e.g. paint already applied in homes, pottery, soil and dust); to educate public health professionals, medical personnel, and the public about the problem and its solutions; and to develop the infrastructure for assessment (including laboratory capacity), surveillance, intervention, evaluation, and treatment.

- *Research* on health education and health promotion appropriate to various cultural settings and "global hot spots" where intervention is urgently needed, and development of country-appropriate surveillance and information management systems.

Silicosis

Silicosis is a well-known fibrogenic lung disease caused by exposure to crystalline quartz silica dust in sandblasting, rock drilling, tunnelling, and other circumstances. WHO estimates that hundreds of thousands of miners and workers engaged in hazardous industrial occupations are currently affected. Exposure to silica can be controlled by the use of substitute agents and dust control measures. Other factors facilitating control include the availability of medical screening and diagnostic tests as well as environmental measuring devices. Effective control has already been demonstrated in some countries. WHO and ILO have announced a global programme for the elimination of occupationally related silicosis.

Key strategies for the elimination of silicosis include the following: substitution of nonhazardous alternatives in abrasive blasting; use of effective engineering devices to suppress dust and provide ventilation; use of effective personal protective equipment when engineering controls do not suffice; periodic monitoring of the work environment for compliance with protective exposure level; and periodic medical surveillance examinations. Research needs include: design and evaluation of health education programmes, training programmes, and technical information for employers and employees; design and testing of economically acceptable engineering controls for local exposure situations; and development of inexpensive methods of real-time exposure measurement and monitoring.

Protein–energy malnutrition

Considering the complex nature of protein–energy malnutrition, the Workgroup could not recommend it as a candidate disease for elimination. However, given its burden in developing countries, a call was made to renew the commitment of governments to further reduce the levels of malnutrition. Indexed by underweight,[a] malnutrition affected 29% of <5-year-olds in developing countries in 1995, a decline of 34% from a decade earlier (*1*).

The group noted that to be successful, programmes must address the multiple causes of malnutrition. The immediate causes are inadequate dietary intake and infection, such as diarrhoeal diseases. Generally, there are problems with both the quantity and quality of foods consumed and these result in multiple deficiencies, notably in energy, protein, and micronutrients such as vitamin A, iodine, iron and zinc. The strategies for preventing malnutrition are well known and include: promoting exclusive breastfeeding for the first 4–6 months of life, and its continuation into the second year; improving complementary feeding of children aged 6–24 months; preventing childhood infections such as diarrhoea which lead to poor nutrient utilization and are a cause of poor appetite; improving the availability of food in the household (food security); providing environmental sanitation and personal hygiene; making health services available; and improving the status and education of women in society.

The group noted that the rates of malnutrition have declined rapidly in countries that have reduced poverty and invested heavily in the social sector (e.g. in health, nutrition, and education). As shown in the developed countries, elimination of malnutrition as a public health problem in developing countries can be attained through sustained and equitable economic growth, increased investments in the social sector, and effective programmes that can reduce malnutrition at an accelerated rate. While much is known about preventing malnutrition in children, there is a need for applied research to improve the effectiveness of nutrition programmes.

Micronutrient malnutrition

The Workgroup noted multiple benefits of addressing several micronutrient deficiencies simultaneously. One particular benefit was increasing the efficiency of delivery. Interactions between micronutrients can facilitate uptake, as in the case where the adequacy of vitamin A improves the utilization of iron. In addition, adequate levels of vitamin A and iron enhance the immune response. In turn, the adequacy of iron reduces the tendency to absorb lead.

---

[a] Underweight is a weight two or more standard deviations below the age- and sex-specific mean in the international reference population used by the U.S. National Center for Health Statistics and WHO. About 2.3% of cases are found below this criterion in the reference curve.

The group noted that the experience of many countries has shown supplementation and fortification of foods to be efficacious and effective in reducing micronutrient deficiencies. The group proposed recommendations for the elimination of four micronutrient deficiencies: iodine deficiency (by the year 2000); vitamin A deficiency (by 2005); iron deficiency (by 2010); and folic-acid-preventable birth defects (by 2005). Key discussion points are summarized in Table 1.

Table 1: **Determinants for the global elimination of selected micronutrient deficiencies**

Determinants	Iodine	Vitamin A	Iron	Folic acid
Reachable target	Eliminate iodine deficiency disease by the year 2005 according to WHO/UNICEF/CCIDD criteria	Eliminate vitamin A deficiency as a public health problem by 2005 according to WHO/UNICEF/CCIDD criteria	Eliminate iron deficiency as a public health problem by 2010	Eliminate folic-acid-preventable birth defects as a public health problem by 2005
Facilitating factors	— Achievable — Methodology available — Remarkable progress — First large-scale fortification programme — Political commitment	— Large-scale supplement coverage integrated with immunization — Multiple ways to increase intake — Large-dose supplements protect children aged 4–6 months — Fortification possible and effective	— Food fortification opportunities — Involvement of private sector	— Evidence that supplemental folic acid prevents a substantial proportion of neural tube defects — Strong observational data that 400 μg folic acid (pteroyl-monoglutamic acid) daily is sufficient — Folic acid baked in grain products works well — Large supplement field trial shown to be effective — Can be combined with other approaches directed to increase consumption of iron and vitamin A and to promote contraceptives
Key strategies	— Iodize salt as the key strategy — Identify and reach those not covered — Develop partnerships for evaluation	— Supplements for children aged 6 months to 5 years as a long-term strategy — Promotion of dietary diversification (e.g. breast-feeding) — Fortification (sugar, oils, processed foods) — Local conditions determine intervention mix	— Supplements as a prevention measure for adolescent girls and schoolchildren and for pregnant women and young children (<2 years) — Fortification; identify appropriate foods for each country — Add iron to foods — Deworm	— Fortify foods — Supplement — Set and monitor goals for levels of blood folate
Research needs	— Develop kits (salt/urine) — Monitor possible side-effects — Improve mixing technologies — Monitor effect on food processing	— Develop simple field assessment tool — Improve quality assurance	*Operational* — Monitor supplement delivery and compliance *Technical* — Assess iron fortification (stability and absorption) — Add iron sprinkles to foods — Fortify condiments (e.g. soy sauce, fish sauce) — Fortify corn flour	— Develop field methods to monitor blood folate status — Develop effective messages for supplement programmes in different cultures

(continued on page 84)

Table 1: **Continued**

Determinants	Iodine	Vitamin A	Iron	Folic acid
Conclusions and recommendations	— Global elimination of iodine deficiency disease as a public health problem is possible — Continued international support is essential to eliminate iodine deficiency disease	— Support and strengthen programmes to eliminate deficiency — Emphasize importance of eliminating vitamin A deficiency to reduce mortality related to infectious diseases — Initiate programmes in countries with high death rates among <5-year-olds — Cover all children with high-dose supplements unless evidence indicates no problem or alternative interventions are in place	— Implement iron deficiency elimination programmes population-wide, focusing on women and young children	— Develop and implement global initiatives to eliminate/prevent folic acid deficiency

The conclusions and recommendations are shown below.

- The achievement of global goals for elimination of iodine deficiency and vitamin A deficiency should be accelerated.

- Based on what is known, programmes should be implemented to eliminate iron deficiency population-wide, with a particular focus on women, young children, and adolescent females.

- Based on what is known, programmes should be implemented to eliminate folic-acid-preventable birth defects as a public health problem, with particular emphasis on adolescent females and women of childbearing age.

- The fact that such programmes might also create opportunities for addressing other micronutrient problems (e.g. zinc and vitamin D deficiencies) should be recognized.

- A major research initiative to demonstrate the efficacy of zinc supplementation/fortification in preventing disease should be undertaken.

- Food fortification with micronutrients represents a major opportunity to cover large populations with multiple micronutrients simultaneously and effectively on a permanent and self-sustaining basis. Involvement of the private food industry as a key partner would enhance the ability to finance this effort through market forces.

- Supplementation represents a major opportunity to join forces with the health sector by synergizing capsule distribution with existing infrastructures such as those required for immunization programmes.

Acknowledgements

Thanks are due to Stephen Corber, William Halperin, Reynaldo Martorell, Shirley Beresford, and Robert Baldwin for their special contributions to this report.

Reference

1. **Administrative Committee on Coordination/Subcommittee on Nutrition (ACC/SCN).** Update on the nutrition situation 1996. *SCN news*, No. 14, July 1997: 7–9.

Report of the Workgroup on Bacterial Diseases

A.R. Hinman[1]

Introduction

The Workgroup felt that 14 factors should be considered when discussing the potential feasibility of elimination or eradication of any disease. These partially overlap but further expand on the seven issues named in the "Framework for considering candidate conditions." The list comprises the following: disease burden; existence of an effective intervention; surveillance/diagnosis mechanism; commonality of delivery; cost-effectiveness; demonstrated effectiveness of the programme; contribution to overall infrastructure; existence of a delivery infrastructure; barriers; roles of technology; existence of nonhuman hosts; time frame; significance of imported cases; and strategies to be followed.

The results of the pre-Conference survey were discussed. The top 10 conditions identified in the survey, in rank order, were as follows: neonatal tetanus; *Haemophilus influenzae* type b (Hib) infection; leprosy; diphtheria; pertussis; tuberculosis (TB); meningococcal disease; congenital syphilis; trachoma; and syphilis. None of these conditions was considered eradicable in the immediate future, although several were thought to be candidates for national or regional elimination.

Several conditions brought up in the survey were deemed important but not currently amenable to elimination or eradication. Consequently, they were not considered further. For diphtheria and pertussis, it was felt there was an incomplete understanding of the epidemiology of the disease and transmission as well as inadequate surveillance systems. Additionally, there was uncertainty as to whether the available interventions could achieve elimination. Meningococcal disease is an important condition for which effective interventions are under development and, in a few years, it may well be a candidate for elimination. The same can be said for pneumococcal disease, which was not included in the top 10 in the survey but is very important because of its high incidence. Regional elimination of typhoid may be feasible but has not been demonstrated. For each of these conditions, improved control is both feasible and necessary.

Subgroups were formed to discuss neonatal tetanus, Hib, TB (and leprosy), and syphilis (both acquired and congenital, with some consideration of chancroid), and trachoma. In the discussions, a continuum of levels of disease incidence was considered, ranging from the situation in which disease occurs uncontrolled to a level of control which, with additional effort, becomes "very good control". The transition from very good control to elimination is likely to require considerable additional effort, in terms of both programme interventions and surveillance. Elimination is a stage which will take major effort to maintain, which will be more difficult the more common the disease is in other parts of the world and the more transmissible it is. In general, elimination should be viewed as a stepping stone to eradication and considered seriously only when eventual eradication seems possible.

Neonatal tetanus

This is a significant problem, with an estimated 490 000 deaths per year (a global rate of 6.5 per 1000 live births). Actions taken to reduce the occurrence of neonatal tetanus would have other positive impacts on health and health care systems, including decreased neonatal mortality and maternal mortality (from other conditions as well as maternal tetanus). Eradication is clearly not feasible, given the ubiquitous distribution of *Clostridium tetani* spores in the soil. Using the strictest definition, elimination also cannot be guaranteed, although radically improved control is possible and should be a high priority. The WHO "elimination" goal of an incidence of <1 per 1000 live births in every district is attainable. Achievement of this goal will require fuller implementation of a three-pronged strategy: vaccination of women of childbearing age, clean delivery, and application of topical antimicrobials to the umbilical stump. The last-mentioned component is not being sufficiently emphasized at present. Because of the combined nature of the strategies, very close collaboration between the Expanded Programme on Immunization (EPI) and Maternal and Child Health (MCH) programmes will be needed to achieve the goal. Since eradication is not feasible and interventions will need to be continued indefinitely, vertical approaches are insufficient; neonatal tetanus control efforts will need to be integrated into developing

[1] The Task Force for Child Survival and Development, One Copenhill, Atlanta, GA 30307, USA.

comprehensive care systems. Substantial research needs remain, from ongoing monitoring of immunity levels in girls attaining childbearing age to development of more effective (possibly single-dose) vaccines.

Haemophilus influenzae type b (Hib) infection

In most parts of the world, the burden of Hib infection has been documented and is of comparable severity. However, in some Western Pacific countries (e.g. China, Republic of Korea, Japan) the severity of this burden is not yet clear. Current estimates are that there are 380 000–600 000 deaths per year globally among under-5-year-olds as a result of Hib infections. Although case management is an important strategy to reduce mortality, it does not have a significant impact on transmission; consequently, the primary intervention is vaccination.

Results from introduction of Hib vaccine have been dramatic in both industrialized and developing countries. The (unexpected) impact of Hib vaccine in reducing carriers of Hib has raised possibilities of elimination/eradication which were previously not considered. In the USA, United Kingdom, and several other industrialized countries, Hib infections have virtually disappeared (>95% reduction) within 4–7 years after introduction of universal vaccination of infants/young children. The disease appears to have been eliminated in Iceland and Finland. In both Chile and the Gambia dramatic results have been seen, and in the latter country there was also a nearly 25% reduction in the incidence of lobar pneumonia among young children following introduction of vaccination. Whether this finding will be replicated in other countries is currently under study. A major barrier to the wider use of Hib vaccine is its current price; at more than US$ 1 per dose, it may not be cost-effective for introduction in developing countries. Fortunately, it appears that the different formulations of Hib vaccine are interchangeable in terms of safety and efficacy. Important research questions include better estimation of the disease burden (especially in south-east Asia), the need to document changes in carrier rates before and after introduction of vaccine, and the impact of infant vaccination on the reservoir of Hib in older age groups. If the disease burden is such as to justify global use of the vaccines and if vaccination has an impact on carrier rates in adults, eradication might be feasible in the relatively near future.

Tuberculosis

Tuberculosis (TB) is currently the leading infectious cause of death in the world, with 2–3 million deaths each year. A three-pronged strategy has been adopted for control of this disease, including case management, vaccination, and preventive therapy. Case management is currently the essential activity of TB control, and the highest priority is given to providing a short course (3–6 months) of directly observed therapy (DOTS) to infectious cases (those with tubercle bacilli demonstrated on microscopic examination of the sputum), with guaranteed supply of drugs. This strategy has been shown to result in high cure rates and is feasible, even in developing countries. BCG vaccination in infancy prevents a substantial proportion of disseminated tuberculosis in children (e.g. TB meningitis), but has little impact on TB transmission or incidence in adults. Preventive therapy, administered to persons who are infected with TB (i.e. tuberculin-positive) but who have not developed disease, is highly effective in preventing development of the disease and is an important strategy to be introduced once a sufficiently high proportion of diagnosed (i.e. infectious) cases are being effectively treated.

The unfortunate interaction between tuberculosis and HIV infection (in which each exacerbates the other) means that the TB problem will deteriorate further in countries which now suffer most from either TB or HIV (e.g. in sub-Saharan Africa and south-east Asia). In addition, multidrug-resistant TB is an increasing problem in many areas, including the Newly Independent States of the Soviet Union and the Russian Federation. Research needs include development of a more effective vaccine, improvements in preventive therapy, better understanding of latent infections and the existence of a possible animal reservoir, and demonstration that elimination is feasible in a defined geographical area. The US "elimination" target of an incidence of <1 case per million population does not meet the Dahlem criteria. Improvements in TB control depend on (and contribute to) general health infrastructure. A long-term (>70 years) goal of elimination/eradication may help retain focus on these efforts.

Leprosy

There are approximately 500 000 new cases of leprosy each year, occurring in geographically restricted areas; 90% of all cases occur in 15 countries. Current interventions focus on finding cases of leprosy and administering directly observed multidrug therapy for 6–24 months (depending on the type of leprosy) and on the use of BCG vaccine. An "elimination" goal has been established, with the target being an incidence of <1 case per 10 000 population. Neither elimination (using Dahlem definitions) nor eradication is feasible, although there are important opportunities for improved control. Some of the barriers to improved control include insufficient knowledge of the epidemiology, pathogenesis, and transmission of leprosy (including carriage and incubation period) and the difficulty in growing the organism in the laboratory.

Syphilis

Approximately 1 million pregnancies each year are complicated by syphilis. Elimination of congenital syphilis in some geographical areas was considered feasible, but not eradication — more because of weaknesses in the health care delivery system than because of faults with the intervention. The same strategies used to attain control and very good control over congenital syphilis should also be adequate to achieve elimination, but with a considerably higher cost. These strategies are as follows: to examine pregnant women at their first prenatal visit, perform an on-site diagnostic test, treat those who are positive and their partners, and take a systematic approach to reduce adult syphilis through diagnosis and treatment of cases of genital ulcer disease. The antenatal care infrastructure necessary for prevention of congenital syphilis is the same as that necessary for prevention of other perinatal conditions such as neonatal tetanus and iron deficiency anaemia. Improvements to the infrastructure will benefit reproductive health services for women overall.

Elimination cannot be achieved strictly through approaches to pregnant women, but also requires activities to prevent and control acquired syphilis in adults. Syndromic approaches to management of genital ulcer disease (primarily syphilis and chancroid) can also have a significant impact on decreasing the transmission of HIV. A goal of "elimination" from the Region of the Americas, which does not meet the Dahlem definition has been established by the Pan American Health Organization. True elimination in the Americas was felt feasible in the next 5–10 years. Elimination of adult syphilis was not considered programmatically feasible at present, although substantial improvements in surveillance and control are both feasible and necessary. It is possible that mass therapy in high prevalence areas could be quite effective in improving control, as it was with yaws. Research needs include development of less invasive diagnostic techniques, effective single-dose oral therapies and vaccines, as well as operational research.

Although elimination of chancroid might be biologically feasible, it does not seem programmatically attainable at present. Factors favouring the potential for elimination include availability of effective oral therapy; clinically apparent, symptomatic disease; a relatively short period of transmissibility; and a high concentration of disease in core transmission groups. Pilot efforts to eliminate chancroid could be undertaken as part of the genital ulcer disease component of congenital syphilis elimination.

Trachoma

Trachoma is the leading preventable cause of blindness worldwide, with an estimated 5.9 million persons blind or at immediate risk because of trichiasis. Trachoma accounts for nearly one-sixth of the global burden of blindness; women are affected disproportionately. Genital strains of *Chlamydia trachomatis* do not infect the eye. Effective interventions have been demonstrated in developing countries to have a major impact on blindness due to trachoma using the "SAFE" strategy — Surgery to correct lid deformity and prevent blindness, Antibiotics for acute infections and community control, Facial hygiene, and Environmental change, including improved access to water and sanitation, and health education.

An "elimination" target of 2020 has been established by an international alliance but does not meet the Dahlem definition. Elimination of blindness due to trachoma is considered feasible; eradication of trachoma is not. Research needs include validation of rapid community assessment techniques, identification of barriers to the acceptance of the preventive surgical procedure, operational research on the effectiveness of annual treatment cycles, and cost–benefit and cost-effectiveness studies.

Conclusions and recommendation

- Each of the above conditions has a significant disease burden, most notably in developing countries.

- Each of these conditions has an effective intervention with at least some existing infrastructure to deliver it, but many of the interventions are not optimal.

- Each condition is poorly controlled globally.

- Each condition has surveillance techniques available, although they may not be in place in all areas.

- None of these conditions is a candidate for eradication in the next 10–15 years with current interventions. Hib infection and congenital syphilis are currently candidates for regional (but not global) elimination. The long-term vision for Hib infection and tuberculosis is eradication (for TB, this would require decades); for congenital syphilis and trachoma the long-term vision is regional elimination.

- Effective control or elimination of most of these conditions requires a combination of strategies, rather than a single strategy such as vaccination.

- Improved control or elimination of each of the conditions is closely related to existing health care delivery systems, rather than a vertical approach. However, it is important that health workers be identified and made responsible for achieving the goals, even though they have many other responsibilities (the concept of "designated" but not "dedicated" personnel).

- Public education and social mobilization are important factors in improved control or elimination/eradication for each of these conditions.

- Behavioural modification is an important factor for the control of most of these conditions.

- There are many research needs for each of the conditions which must be addressed before eradication could be attempted. These range from the need for improved understanding of the epidemiology of disease to developing improved interventions and improved strategies to deliver interventions.

- Elimination is expensive, both in the extra effort needed to achieve zero incidence and in the surveillance system needed to document zero incidence.

- Unless elimination is a step on the road to eradication, very good control may be a more appropriate goal. This would potentially allow broader use of the additional resources which may be required for elimination.

- Public health institutions have been imprecise in their use of the term "elimination", often using it to indicate very good control (e.g. "elimination as a public health problem"). Several incidence goals have been set and labelled as elimination goals which do not meet the definitions agreed at the Dahlem Workshop. Efforts should be made to use this term precisely. None the less, it is important to set specific targets for control activities ("control with a goal"), which could encompass some of the targets currently labelled as "elimination" (e.g. global goal for neonatal tetanus, U.S. goal for tuberculosis).

Given all these factors, the Workgroup recommends that, while actively pursuing the research needed to improve our understanding of these diseases and our interventions for dealing with them, the global community should take aggressive action to improve global control of neonatal tetanus, *Haemophilus influenzae* type b infection, tuberculosis, leprosy, congenital syphilis, and trachoma.

Acknowledgements

Thanks are due to Helen Makela and Suriadi Gunawan (Co-Chairs), and to Ken Castro, Joe Cook, Lyn Finelli, Dace Madore and Rebecca Prevots (subgroup rapporteurs) for their special contribution to this report.

Report of the Workgroup on Parasitic Diseases

J.P. Figueroa[1]

Introduction

The Workgroup reviewed and agreed to work with the definitions of control, elimination and eradication published in the Dahlem Workshop Report. However, it was noted that a number of resolutions of regional and international bodies, including WHO, PAHO, and the World Bank, included the expression "elimination [of a particular disease] as a public health problem".

The criteria for assessing the eradicability of diseases and conditions given in the Dahlem Workshop Report were accepted by the group. It was noted that the development of an effective strategy was part of demonstrating the feasibility of elimination. The economic impact or benefit of disease elimination/eradication may be with respect to intervention factors, including cost-effectiveness, equity (distribution issues), and the impact on the economy. The list of candidate parasitic diseases was reviewed and the group concluded that dracunculiasis was eradicable at present with current tools; separate working subgroups were designated to consider onchocerciasis, lymphatic filariasis, Chagas disease, and "other parasites".

Caution was expressed in relation to the capacity of many developing countries to engage in more than a very limited number of eradication/elimination campaigns at a given time. There is already a global eradication campaign for poliomyelitis and for candidate diseases such as measles, and there are a number of regional disease elimination campaigns. Candidate diseases for elimination will need to be ranked in order of priority on a global and regional basis. In addition, issues of certification of disease elimination and eradication need to be considered. For example, the ability of parasites to survive for long periods in humans makes the certification of elimination even more difficult.

Onchocerciasis

It was agreed that onchocerciasis was a strong candidate for elimination as a public health problem, but not for eradication at the present time. As such, the subgroup endorsed the recommendations and defini-tion used by the 1993 International Task Force for Disease Elimination, where the term "elimination as a public health problem" was used. This is a concept that encompasses both global control and elimination of infection in selected areas.

Essential facilitating factors

Considerable achievements have been made towards elimination of onchocerciasis in most of the Americas, all countries within the Onchocerciasis Control Programme in West Africa (OCP), and in several other African countries. Progressive increase in treatment with ivermectin has been achieved, with 500 000 doses of treatment having been distributed in 1988 and 18 million in 1997. This represents near complete coverage in the OCP and the Americas, and about 33% coverage in the APOC (African Programme for Onchocerciasis Control) countries. Extensive partnerships exist which are dedicated to the goal of sustained and complete global ivermectin treatment; the partners include Merck & Co., WHO, the World Bank, Inter-American Development Bank, nongovernmental organizations, research institutes, ministries of health, other donors, and the endemic communities.

Constraining factors

An important constraining factor is that ivermectin is not effective in killing the adult worms (macrofilariae). Other factors are the difficulty in achieving and maintaining a sufficiently high coverage and treatment frequency to interrupt transmission, the long life span of the adult worms, and active human and vector migration.

Key strategies

Annual or semiannual mass ivermectin treatment must be sustained through community-based distribution programmes in endemic areas.

Research needs

- Surveillance: epidemiological assessment and mapping; tools, techniques, and strategies to monitor the effectiveness of interventions; and criteria for interruption of transmission.

[1] Chief Medical Officer, Ministry of Health, Kingston, Jamaica.

- Diagnosis: PCR/DNA probes for detection of *Onchocerca* larvae in blackflies.

- Other: development of community-level strategies to ensure programme sustainability; assessment of the effect of long-term exposure to ivermectin on longevity/fecundity in the adult worm; development of new drugs (macro- and microfilaricides); monitoring the emergence of drug resistance (especially to ivermectin); monitoring the impact of fly and human migration patterns on the programme; and assessment of the social and economic impact of the programme.

Conclusions

- Onchocerciasis can be eliminated as a public health problem, as has been demonstrated in the Americas and OCP.

- At present, onchocerciasis cannot be considered as a candidate for eradication. This position may need to be reconsidered in a period of 5–10 years on the basis of the data on the long-term effect of mass treatment on transmission.

Lymphatic filariasis

Goals and strategies

- *Goal I.* Reduce microfilaraemia to interrupt transmission and prevent infection. (In areas of subperiodic Brugian infections (<5% of lymphatic filariasis cases), the goal is limited to decreasing transmission and reducing the incidence of infection. Strategies to achieve this goal included the following: mass treatment for 4–6 years of entire at-risk populations with two-drug regimens (choosing among diethylcarbamazine (DEC), ivermectin, and albendazole); use of salt fortified with DEC for 1–4 years; and vector control as an adjunctive measure.

- *Goal II.* Alleviate and reduce the suffering of persons with filaria-related disease. Strategies to achieve this goal include the following: community-based care and training which emphasizes hygiene and other simple measures to prevent the occurrence of acute attacks and to reverse the changes due to lymphoedema and elephantiasis; and health education.

Essential facilitating factors

- Transmission of the parasite is inefficient.

- The parasite does not reproduce in the vector.

- There is no animal reservoir for *Wuchereria bancrofti* or nocturnal Brugia infections; although animal reservoirs for subperiodic *Brugia malayi* (causing <5% of lymphatic filariasis) do exist, they are of uncertain importance for human infections.

- Simple, rapid, accurate tools exist for diagnosis; although no antigen detection assay is currently available for *B. malayi*, there are highly sensitive, but more labour-intensive, PCR diagnostic techniques.

- Treatment to reduce and suppress microfilarial levels in blood is effective, inexpensive, safe, simple and suitable for large-scale mass treatment (i.e. in an annual single-dose regimen). A variety of treatment options (i.e. drugs and drug combinations) are available, reducing the likelihood of the development of parasite resistance to a single drug. Treatment with these drugs provides collateral health benefits, including a reduction in the burden of intestinal helminth infections (and, with ivermectin, relief from scabies and lice infestations); this feature enhances the programme's acceptability and integration with other health programmes.

- Treatment for filaria-associated disease leading to prevention of the debilitating acute attacks and reversibility of lymphoedema and elephantiasis is simple, uses appropriate technology, can be carried out at the community level, and can provide collateral benefits for community development.

- In filariasis-endemic areas, the disease is regarded as one of high importance, in part because of its disfiguring clinical manifestations.

- Several countries already have national filariasis elimination activities underway, and others have new national plans of action.

- Partners from the private sector have already expressed a strong commitment to filariasis elimination, as exemplified by the drug donation by SmithKline Beecham.

- The type of Brugian filariasis, for which an animal reservoir may sometimes exist and for which diagnostic tools are less well developed, accounts for <5% of all lymphatic filariasis cases worldwide.

Research needs

- Simplified diagnostic tools for *B. malayi* infection.

- Definition of the importance of the animal reservoir for *B. malayi*.

- Development of means to monitor for emergence of drug resistance.

- Development of means for integrating the twin goals of interrupting transmission through mass treatment and relieving suffering through community-based care.

- Surveillance: epidemiological assessment and mapping; means for monitoring the effectiveness of interventions in reducing and interrupting transmission; and criteria for certification of elimination of infection.

- Determination of the criteria required to initiate mass treatment, the duration of programmes, and whether there is a threshold of microfilariae prevalence below which transmission cannot be sustained.

- Assessment of the efficacy of different drugs, drug combinations, and annual sequences of drugs against the adult worm and microfilariae.

- Estimation of the costs and benefits of mass treatment with antifilarial drugs and drug combinations.

- Development of models of programme implementation, and determining the optimal approach for integrating these with primary health care and other health care services.

- Development of more effective macrofilaricidal approaches for treating the individual patient.

- Development of means for measuring, increasing, and sustaining compliance at the community level.

Conclusions

- *W. bancrofti* and periodic *B. malayi* infection, which cause more than 95% of lymphatic filariasis, can be eliminated and potentially are eradicable.

- Infection with *B. malayi* can be eliminated except in those foci where animal reservoirs exist for the "subperiodic" form of this parasite. Additional research is required to establish whether or not this infection in animals is important as a source of infections in humans.

Chagas disease

Elimination of *Triatoma infestans* — the main domestic vector of Chagas disease in the Southern Cone Region — is an attainable goal, except in some areas of Bolivia, where sylvatic foci of this species exist. From the beginning of national programmes in

Uruguay and Brazil in 1980, *T. infestans* has been eliminated in >95% of the municipalities that were formerly infested. In the places or regions where Chagas disease (CD) programmes were well implemented (as reflected by quality and continuity), there was a dramatic decrease in human CD cases and the interruption of transmission whenever the level of house infestations decreased to 3% or less. In addition, serological surveys showed an impact on schoolchildren: for example, in Brazil (São Paulo State) and Uruguay, there were substantial declines in seropositivity in schoolchildren from the 1960s to 1995. Changes also occurred in other groups, including blood donors in Brazil (in 1979, 5% were seropositive versus 0.7% in 1995); pregnant women in Bambui (in 1954, >45% were seropositive, compared with 18% in 1963, 1.5% in 1990, and 0% in 1997). Based on the experience in the Southern Cone countries, the subgroup concluded that domiciliary Chagas disease could probably be eliminated as a human infection in most regions.

Essential facilitating factors

- The primary vectors are susceptible to many insecticides and are reduced by improved housing.

- Transmission is slow and difficult.

- Effective control tools are available.

- Control programmes (especially in Brazil and Uruguay) have demonstrated the feasibility of elimination.

Constraining factors

Constraining factors include the existence of multiple vectors, some of which are not domiciliary, and of multiple animal reservoirs; the lack of political will in some countries; the absence of an effective vaccine or drug against chronic infection; and a complex strategy requiring six complementary interventions.

Key strategies

- Preliminary assessment of the problem, including vector mapping, serological testing, and (in the initial stages) clinical testing which requires good laboratory support.

- Epidemiological surveillance to be conducted with the effective participation of the community.

- Health education and community mobilization.

- Insecticides for vector control.

- Housing improvement.

Table 1: **Evaluation of additional candidate diseases based on Dahlem criteria**[a]

Candidate disease	Epidemiological vulnerability	Effective practical intervention	Demonstration of feasibility	Burden of disease	Expected cost of eradication	Synergy of eradication efforts	Necessity of eradication over control	Total score
Malaria	1	1	1–3	3	1	3	3	13–15
Taeniasis/ cysticercosis	3	3	2	1	2–3	3	1	15–16
Visceral leishmaniasis	2	1	1	1–2	1	2	1–2	9–11
Schistosomiasis	1–3	2	1	3	1	3	1	12–14
Geohelminth diseases	1	2–3	1	3	2–3	3	1	13–15
Echinococcosis	1–2	1–2	2	1–2	2	1	1	9–12
Fascioliasis	1–2	1–2	1	1	1–2	1	1	7–10

[a] Key:
1 = poor candidate for eradication/elimination.
2 = average candidate for eradication/elimination.
3 = good candidate for eradication/elimination.

- Routine screening of blood bank blood should be instituted in endemic countries; blood should be treated before use if the disease incidence is >10%.

- Congenital cases need to be identified and treated.

Research needs

- Development of a simple, cheap, rapid blood test with high sensitivity and specificity

- KAP studies to guide health education/community mobilization interventions.

- Vector studies to a) determine to what extent and why sylvatic species infest peri-domestic environments, and b) develop methods of vector detection when vector population densities are low.

- Continued development of drugs for curing chronic infection.

- Determination of the efficacy of treatment of chronic infection with currently available drugs.

- Operational studies of housing improvement methods.

- Assessment of *Trypanosoma cruzi* strains responsible for human and nonhuman animal reservoir infections.

Other parasitic diseases

The Subgroup on Other Parasitic Diseases considered seven parasitic diseases using the criteria identified by the Dahlem Workshop (Table 1). The diverse nature of the infectious agents (protozoa and helminths) and their modes of transmission (e.g. vectorborne, soil-transmitted, foodborne and zoonotic) makes comparison of these diseases difficult. Many of these infections, in their natural habitats, are not considered susceptible to elimination using current technologies. However, experience has revealed that they are capable of elimination from certain areas to which they have spread or been introduced.

Malaria

Previous attempts to eradicate malaria were unsuccessful. However, the extreme burden imposed by this disease warrants that it continue to be considered for elimination. Further research is essential for developing a better understanding of the disease and its effective intervention.

Taeniasis/cysticercosis

Taenia solium taeniasis/cysticercosis was considered to be potentially eradicable. The two-host life-cycle of this cestode, including humans and domestic pigs makes it vulnerable to a variety of interventions. Historical experiences in western Europe indicate that this infection may even disappear without targeted interventions. Pigs, which rarely are allowed to survive past one year, are an excellent focal point for surveillance of the infection which may be done by local people without expensive equipment or training. There are rapid diagnostic tests for the infective stages in both humans and pigs, and effective and inexpensive drugs for mass treatment of intestinal tapeworm infections in humans. There is a need to demonstrate the cost-effectiveness and sustainability of intervention strategies in a variety of endemic situations.

Visceral leishmaniasis

The leishmaniases are difficult to eliminate because of the existence of reservoirs in domestic and wild animals. However, there are "anthropophilic" strains/species that are vulnerable to elimination by effective vector control and targeted treatment. Current epidemics of these strains are occurring in Sudan, Bangladesh and parts of India. There is a need for demonstration projects to determine the possible effectiveness of such measures.

Schistosomiasis

Schistosomiasis is difficult to control under most situations. However, its public health burden makes it necessary to consider new approaches to elimination. The availability of an inexpensive and highly effective drug, praziquantel, provides a tool for greatly reducing morbidity and rates of transmission in endemic areas.

Geohelminth diseases

The geohelminths (ascaris, hookworms and whipworms) currently infect about one-quarter to one-third of the world's population, causing impairment of growth and cognitive development of infected children. Although refractory to elimination in most areas, mass treatment of school-age children is increasingly seen as a cost-effective intervention strategy for reducing the associated morbidity and developmental problems in affected populations. Such interventions are well accepted and form the basis for other community health interventions.

Echinococcosis

The zoonotic helminth *Echinococcus granulosus*, which causes human hydatid disease, is widely prevalent in populations involved in raising sheep and some other livestock animals. The disease has been effectively eliminated from island and regional situations by reduction in the number and/or by treatment of dogs, the definitive host of the tapeworm. The existence of sylvatic cycles of *Echinococcus* spp. precludes eradication of the agent. Similarly, with fascioliasis, the existence of animal reservoirs precludes eradication; however, improved drug therapy provides effective treatment of the disease in humans and animals.

Recommendations

Definitions

• International agencies should review with other stakeholders the definitions and use of the terms "elimination of infection and disease" with a view to achieving a consensus.

Research

• Funding agencies should promote research to identify an effective macrofilaricide for onchocerciasis.

• Endpoints for use in the certification of the eventual elimination/eradication of parasitic diseases need to be determined.

Acknowledgement

Thanks are due to David Addiss, Joel Breman, Dan Colley, Emanuel Miri, P.R. Narayanan, Peter Ndumbe, Eric Ottesen, Frank Richards, Peter Schantz, and Craig Withers for their special contributions to this report.

References

1. **Blanks J et al.** The Onchocerciasis Elimination Program for the Americas: a history of partnership. *Pan American journal of public health*, 1998, **3**: 367–374.
2. **Centres for Disease Control and Prevention.** Recommendations of the International Task Force for Disease Eradication. *Morbidity and mortality weekly report, recommendations and reports*, 1993, **42** (RR-16).
3. **Dowdle WR, Hopkins DR. eds.** The eradication of infectious diseases: report of the Dahlem Workshop on the Eradication of Infections Diseases. Chichester, John Wiley & Sons, 1998.
4. **Duke BOL.** Onchocerciasis (river blindness) — can it be eradicated? *Parasitology today*, 1990, **6**: 82–84.
5. **Schantz PM et al.** Potential eradicability of taeniasis and cysticercosis. *Bulletin of the Pan American Health Organization*, 1993, **27**: 397–403.
6. *Control of Chagas disease. Report of a WHO Expert Committee.* Geneva, World Health Organization, 1991 (WHO Technical Report Series, No. 811).
7. Four TDR diseases can be "eliminated". *TDR News*, 1996, **49**: 7–11.
8. *Lymphatic filariasis: the disease and its control. Fifth report of the WHO Expert Committee on Filariasis.* Geneva, World Health Organization, 1992 (WHO Technical Report Series, No. 821).
9. *Onchocerciasis and its control. Report of a WHO Expert Committee on Onchocerciasis Control.* Geneva, World Health Organization, 1995 (WHO Technical Report Series, No. 852).

Report of the Workgroup on Viral Diseases

J. Losos[1]

Introduction

The Workgroup identified measles, rubella, and viral hepatitis B as priority candidates for eradication. Viral hepatitis A is not recommended for elimination or eradication at the present time. Yellow fever, rabies, and Japanese encephalitis cannot be eradicated because they are found in animal reservoirs, but they can be controlled, in some cases to the point of elimination, through immunization programmes.

The group used the definitions of eradication and elimination adopted by the Dahlem Workshop on the Eradication of Infectious Diseases. Elimination refers to reducing the incidence of a disease to zero within a defined geographical area, with continued intervention measures as needed, while eradication refers to permanently reducing the incidence of a disease to zero worldwide, with no intervention measures required.

Viral hepatitis A and B

Viral hepatitis A

Hepatitis A virus (HAV) infects more than 80% of the population of many developing countries by late adolescence, and is common in developed countries as well (1–3). It produces a generally asymptomatic infection in under-5-year-olds, and an acute, self-limited disease in older children, adolescents, and adults (1, 4).

Inactivated HAV vaccines, which only became commercially available in 1994, effectively confer protection in more than 95% of vaccinated persons (2, 5, 6). Routine vaccination of children aged >2 years has effectively interrupted community-wide epidemics, and sustained vaccination has eliminated transmission of infection in these communities. While the potential for elimination of HAV exists, it cannot be recommended at this time, because of the impeding factors discussed below.

Essential facilitating factors. Routine childhood immunization with an effective, cell-culture-derived,

inactive HAV vaccine has been shown to be cost-effective in populations with high rates of infection. The administration of the vaccine during community-wide outbreaks has been shown to be effective in interrupting transmission of the virus. The vaccine can also be administered with other vaccines and combined with other vaccine antigens (2).

Essential impeding factors. HAV vaccine is expensive, making large-scale purchases by developing countries difficult. Also, there is no vaccine formulation or schedule for use in infancy and early childhood, and it cannot be included in the Expanded Programme for Immunization (EPI).

Key strategies. It will be important to demonstrate the feasibility of eliminating HAV transmission in specific geographical areas. National acute disease surveillance must be improved to better differentiate viral hepatitis A from viral hepatitis B.

Research needs. Two areas of research are immediate priorities:

— development of decision/economic models for hepatitis A vaccination in developing countries; and

— development of vaccine formulations and schedules for infants and children <2 years old.

Conclusions and recommendations. These are as follows:

— eradication of HAV transmission appears to be both biologically and epidemiologically feasible;

— the time required to achieve cessation of transmission may be short;

— the coupling of HAV immunization with other vaccines appears to be feasible; and

— population-based projects to demonstrate sustained elimination of HAV transmission should be initiated as early as possible.

Viral hepatitis B

Viral hepatitis B (HBV), which affects an estimated 360 million people worldwide, is a primary candidate for elimination or eradication. It occurs most often in Africa, the Pacific Islands, part of South America, most of Asia, and in ethnically defined populations

[1] Assistant Deputy Minister, Health Protection Branch, Health Canada, Ottawa, Ontario, Canada.

in Australia, New Zealand, and the USA (7). Chronic infection, which usually begins in early childhood, is associated with risk of death from chronic liver disease, primarily as an adult, and with the risk of liver cancer, a leading cause of death among many adults in developing countries. These consequences generally develop among adults at the most productive times in their lives, creating a high economic burden worldwide.

Essential facilitating factors. Pre- and post-exposure immunization can prevent infection. Limited population-based studies have demonstrated that new infection can be prevented, resulting in a marked reduction in the chronic carrier state among routinely immunized cohorts of children. Progress towards ending transmission of the virus can be measured by the reduction in chronic viral hepatitis B infection within immunized cohorts in a geographic area.

HBV vaccine can be used in combination with other vaccines given to infants and children. High levels of infant immunization, beginning at a time that would prevent perinatal transmission (e.g. first dose at birth), may ultimately lead to global elimination of HBV transmission.

The framework for eliminating HBV transmission already exists. Nongovernmental organizations and voluntary health organizations interested in preventing viral hepatitis and HBV-related hepatotocellular carcinoma hepatitis can facilitate broader prevention partnerships, while practical diagnostic tools to detect infection are available commercially to both developed and developing countries. Many countries have demonstrated their commitment to eliminating HBV transmission by including the hepatitis B vaccine in the EPI.

Essential impeding factors. The cost per dose of hepatitis B vaccine is relatively high, preventing many poorer countries from including it in their EPI. However, significant cost reductions have been achieved through combined regional vaccine purchases. More seriously, while HBV transmission can be eliminated among immunized people, immunizations would have to be maintained for several generations for eradication to be achieved, because of the virus's persistence in chronically infected persons who did not benefit from immunization.

Key strategies. Routine immunization of infants through EPI is crucial, with vaccination beginning at a time that will prevent perinatal transmission. Immunizations near birth would have the subsidiary benefit of strengthening maternal and child health

programmes and promoting the use of trained birth attendants. Current acute disease surveillance systems should be strengthened to identify the etiology of acute and chronic hepatitis, including HBV infection.

Research needs. The following are priority areas for research:

— development of economic models which can be used to convince policy-makers of the need for hepatitis B immunization;

— improvements in vaccines, including the development of vaccines which require fewer doses while providing long-term immune memory, or which are administered orally; and

— determination of HBV variations which may be resistant to vaccine-induced antibody.

Conclusion and recommendation. Hepatitis B immunization should become a component of EPI in all countries, with a vaccination schedule that maximizes the likelihood of eliminating transmission of HBV infection.

Measles

Highly contagious and easily transmitted, measles is responsible for fully 10% of deaths from all causes among <5-year-olds (8). It is the eighth leading cause of death worldwide, being responsible for an estimated one million deaths each year, or 2.7% of disability-adjusted life years in 1990 (9).

The availability of an effective vaccine which produces ≥85% immunity after one dose administered at 9 months of age, and ≥95% immunity after two doses (10), the fact that humans are thought to be the only reservoir capable of sustaining transmission, and the successful control of measles in the Americas make measles the next likely candidate for eradication. However, its highly contagious nature and the ease with which it can be imported from endemic areas by air travel mean that eradicating measles will require a coordinated global effort over a relatively short period of time. Global coverage with one dose of measles vaccine was estimated at 81% in 1996 (11). Two regions have already set a measles-elimination goal — by the year 2000 for the Region of the Americas and 2010 for the Eastern Mediterranean Region. The European Region will be considering this year whether to set the same goal for 2007. China and several southern African and Pacific island countries have embarked on accelerated approaches for measles control or elimination.

Essential facilitating factors. Strategies developed in the Americas have demonstrated that it is technically feasible to interrupt measles transmission in a large area for a variable time period. However, it remains essential that the use of similar strategies demonstrate the same impact in other regions of the world. The experience gained and lessons learned from the poliomyelitis eradication programme will greatly facilitate the implementation of measles eradication, particularly with respect to political support, donor coordination, private sector involvement, and surveillance strategies.

Essential inhibiting factors. A weak health infrastructure in developing countries will inhibit the eradication of measles, which requires substantial effort and resources; in developed countries, the disease has not been perceived as a priority so that adequate efforts to control or eliminate it have not been made. Both of these factors pose a risk for those countries that have eliminated transmission, and they will have to sustain high levels of effort to ensure high immunity and careful surveillance. In addition, the safety of injections during campaigns and routine immunizations can be an issue if sufficient care is not taken.

Key strategies. The approach to measles eradication should be implemented in phases; the initial focus should be on elimination of the disease in the industrialized world, where both infrastructure and resources for elimination are readily available. This means fostering interest in measles elimination in the developed countries, while accelerating worldwide control of the disease, especially in those areas at high risk of measles mortality.

It will be important to capitalize on the experience of different regions of the world. For example, strategies developed and implemented by PAHO — such as the one-time mass campaign (catch-up), the achievement and sustaining of a high measles coverage level among each cohort of newborns (keep-up), and periodic campaigns to prevent accumulation of susceptible individuals (follow-up) — have interrupted transmission of measles over a prolonged period in many countries. Surveillance measures can be built on existing acute flaccid paralysis (AFP) surveillance developed for the poliomyelitis eradication programme.

Research needs. Priority areas for research include the following:

— study of changes in the patterns of transmission with increasing immunization levels, especially in adult populations, and development of method-ologies for the evaluation of the build-up of susceptibility in different age groups to guide strategy selection;

— characterization of the immunobiology of measles virus infection and immunization;

— examination of alternative routes for administering the vaccine, including safety issues, and alternative methods of immunization at an earlier age;

— the need to develop adequate indicators for evaluating surveillance and documenting the impact of intervention; and

— development of a rapid diagnostic assay for field use.

Conclusions and recommendations. These are shown below.

• It is biologically plausible to eradicate measles with the present vaccine. In the Americas, measles transmission appears to have been interrupted in many countries for variable time intervals, but elimination has yet to be demonstrated in other regions.

• Measles elimination is technically feasible in developed countries, which should proceed with elimination as a step towards global eradication.

• In other countries, accelerating measles control should be the priority, especially in areas with high mortality.

• Experience from regional and country interventions should be used to refine the strategies for eventual eradication.

• Any consideration for elimination or eradication of measles should not jeopardize the poliomyelitis eradication effort.

• Countries undertaking measles elimination should incorporate measles surveillance into their poliomyelitis surveillance systems, including the poliomyelitis laboratory network.

Rubella

Rubella generally presents as a mild or asymptomatic infection in adults and children. In pregnant women, however, especially in the first trimester, rubella infection can result in stillbirth, miscarriage, or the constellation of birth defects known as congenital rubella syndrome (CRS) (12). The most commonly described CRS anomalies include nerve deafness, cataracts, cardiac anomalies, impaired intrauterine growth, inflammatory lesions of different organs, and mental retardation.

Rubella is endemic in most countries of the world. In the absence of major epidemics, it has been estimated that more than 20 000 infants are born with CRS each year in the Americas, and at least 236 000 cases in each nonepidemic year in developing countries. Approximately 30% of suspected measles cases in the English-speaking Caribbean and Mexico were laboratory confirmed as rubella. Eradicating rubella with the present vaccine is biologically plausible. However many other issues must first be addressed, including the marginal cost of adding rubella to measles eradication, and the determination of the best strategies to interrupt transmission (*13*).

Essential facilitating factors. Humans are the only known reservoir for rubella. Also, a highly effective rubella vaccine exists, and can be delivered in combination with the measles vaccine, leading to potential economic gains in health costs.

Essential inhibiting factors. The global burden of rubella and CRS remains undefined in many developing countries. However, in the absence of high coverage with the vaccine, there is a potential risk of CRS because of susceptible women not having been immunized or exposed to wild rubella during childhood. As a result, high levels of routine immunization must be maintained. Finally, depending on the vaccination programme implemented, there exists a potential risk for the age of infection to shift to older age groups.

Key strategies. The first step towards elimination or eradication of rubella is to gather data on the virus, by building epidemiological and laboratory surveillance for rubella in conjunction with the measles surveillance system, and by establishing a surveillance system for CRS. Owing to the different epidemiology of rubella, the target age groups to be immunized will need to be wider, and will need to include additional intervention in adults.

Research needs. Priorities for research include the following:

— determining the burden of CRS in developing countries;

— investigating the risk of shifting the age of infection to older age groups and the need to cover a wider target age group (other than young children) to interrupt transmission;

— developing a combined measles/rubella laboratory field test;

— establishing demonstration projects to show that rubella can be eliminated, and that elimination can be sustained in certain countries; and

— conducting studies of the epidemiology of rubella transmission in developing countries, particularly the role of adults in transmission.

Conclusions and recommendations. These are as follows:

• Countries undertaking measles elimination should add rubella vaccine to their measles vaccination programme as a way to improve control of rubella and as part of a sustainable national immunization programme.

• In these countries, rubella surveillance should be incorporated into the measles surveillance programme and CRS surveillance systems should be established.

• Countries wishing to control CRS rapidly should immunize women of childbearing age as part of a sustainable national immunization programme.

• Countries which implement routine childhood immunization should also make efforts to immunize susceptible women of childbearing age through programmes such as postpartum vaccination to prevent CRS.

Yellow fever and other zoonotic diseases

Yellow fever

Yellow fever, a mosquito-borne viral disease, is not considered eradicable at the present time. However, an excellent and inexpensive vaccine exists, and its sustained use regionally has led to effective control of the disease and elimination of recognized outbreaks (*14, 15*). The threat of introduction of yellow fever to Asia carries an urgency beyond its local impact in Africa and South America, and control of the disease deserves priority (*16*).

Essential facilitating factors. While there are major differences in disease epidemiology in South America and Africa, the yellow fever vaccine, which has a long history of safe and effective use, protects against all strains of the virus (*14*). It is heat stable, confers long-term immunity after a single dose, and, in limited studies, has been given with other vaccines, including measles and meningococcal vaccines, without interference. The vaccine can be produced in several countries where there is a risk of transmission, and highly specific international standards for vaccine production and quality have been delineated and promulgated.

Essential impeding factors. Sylvatic yellow fever in South America leads to sporadic cases and small outbreaks of the disease; focused immunization programmes may be effective and sufficient for control. In some areas, the vaccine has been incorporated into local EPI programmes. However, because outbreaks occur sporadically and in remote areas, it is politically difficult to justify the resources for universal coverage. This current inability to implement universal immunization at the present time complicates the vaccination programme. The real risk in South America is that of urban epidemics, as most urban centres have been reinfected by *Aedes aegypti* mosquitos, the principal transmitter of urban yellow fever (*17, 18*). Rapid spread from South America by air travel could mean an increased risk of urban yellow fever in Asia and the Pacific (*16*).

In Africa, the burden of disease is comprised of both endemic transmission and epidemics (*19, 20*). With few exceptions, vaccination programmes have not been initiated or maintained, owing to the lack of national resources and political will to sustain immunization programmes (*21*). The disease is a low priority because it occurs only in intermittent epidemics and mainly in rural areas, where it is less visible and has less political impact. Epidemiological assessments of the incidence and burden of the disease are also poor.

The relatively low volume of vaccine use prevents a reduction in vaccine costs and inhibits manufacturers from developments that could facilitate public health implementation, such as the formulation of combination vaccines. For example, development of a measles–yellow fever combination vaccine was initiated with WHO's encouragement by Pasteur–Mérieux–Connaught in 1984, but was discontinued in 1992 when implementation of yellow fever vaccine in African EPI programmes did not evolve as expected.

Key strategies. Yellow fever is found in animal reservoirs, and therefore is not considered eradicable at the present time. However, wider use of a vaccine could control and effectively eliminate the disease. This could be accomplished by including yellow fever vaccine in the EPI programmes of African countries at risk and implementing catch-up immunization, as recommended by WHO and UNICEF, immunizing selected groups of people at high risk of sylvatic yellow fever in South America, intensifying surveillance and immunization in areas at high risk for urban epidemics, and strengthening enforcement of international travel and vaccination requirements to prevent the spread of yellow fever to Asia.

Research needs. Priority areas for research include the following:

— improving disease burden estimates in Africa, especially a better assessment of the burden due to endemic transmission, as well as quantitative data on the incidence and economic costs of the disease and the costs of not taking preventive measures;

— establishing national and regional diagnostic laboratories to improve surveillance, and developing a diagnostic kit suitable for field use to facilitate surveillance in rural areas;

— developing yellow fever combination vaccines that will facilitate the inclusion of the vaccine in routine and catch-up immunization programmes;

— developing a greater understanding of the immunogenicity and safety of yellow fever vaccine in HIV-infected persons, including the potential for delayed vaccine clearance and subsequent transmission.

Conclusions and recommendations. These are as follows:

• Yellow fever virus is not considered eradicable; however, the availability of a vaccine of unparalleled safety and efficacy argues for its wider use to control and, effectively, to eliminate the disease. Barriers to its control are not due to scientific or technical limitations, but to administrative and economic considerations of health care delivery.

• In Africa, vaccine implementation has been inhibited by the perception of low public health priority and the absence of sufficient public will to sustain routine childhood immunization. Improved surveillance and quantification of the economic costs of the disease are needed to stimulate nongovernmental and governmental organizations into action.

• As a first step, obstacles to the implementation of the 1988 joint WHO/UNICEF recommendation to include yellow fever vaccine in African EPI programmes should be identified with a view to overcoming these barriers. A WHO technical consensus meeting, held on 3–4 March 1998, addressed these issues.

Rabies

Rabies is not considered eradicable at present. By controlling the infection in animal reservoirs, however, the disease can be controlled in humans as well (22–24). This will result in reduced human mortality due to rabies and reduced human morbidity and economic costs of post-exposure prophylaxis.

Essential facilitating factors. Because the burden of disease is primarily in urban areas (25), where dogs constitute the principal animal reservoir, control of rabies is more feasible, and has been demonstrated in many areas, most recently in Latin America. Rabies control in its wild animal reservoirs has achieved some measure of success, particularly in red foxes in western Europe and eastern Canada, through distribution of oral baited vaccines (26). Because of innate biological and ecological differences in reservoir species, however, further advances will require strategies to be specifically tailored for each reservoir.

Public awareness of the risks of rabies also facilitates control programmes, as does the wide availability of vaccines for both veterinary and human use. Epizootiological and epidemiological surveillance is facilitated by viral antigenic and genomic markers (27) associated with reservoir hosts.

Essential impeding factors. Effective control of rabies requires partnership between departments of health and agriculture, agencies responsible for environmental health and wildlife protection, and the private sector (23). Overlapping responsibilities among government agencies necessitate close coordination.

An essential component of effective rabies post-exposure prophylaxis includes rabies immune globulin, which is frequently in short supply and too costly for routine use in many developing countries. Licensed cell-culture-based vaccines are available for veterinary and human use.

Key strategies. A combination of dog control and immunization is the key to controlling urban rabies, as is the use of oral vaccine in baits to control or reduce sylvatic rabies transmission (26, 28, 29). Programmes to limit human exposure to animal bites should be promoted. Access to post-exposure prophylaxis should be made more available. Humans at high risk for rabies, such as veterinarians, persons with vocational risks, and members of certain occupational groups, should be immunized prior to exposure (23, 24). Continued development and evaluation of oral vaccination, as an adjunct to traditional control measures, should be encouraged.

Research needs. Priorities for research include the following:

— developing a safe and effective vaccine for mass immunization of dogs, such as an oral bait vaccine (26), which does not pose a threat of inadvertent ingestion by children;

— replacing brain-derived vaccines, which cause neurological reactions, with existing cell-culture based vaccines (24);

— ensuring the safety and efficacy of currently manufactured rabies vaccines, since, in some instances, production and quality in many developing countries are not well controlled (28);

— identifying less costly, effective alternatives to human rabies immune globulin (30);

— developing a better understanding of all aspects of rabies transmission in bats, which has emerged as the most important cause of rabies in the USA (30) and the only recognized native rabies reservoir in Australia (31);

— exploiting existing knowledge of the virology of rhabdoviruses to develop safe and effective antiviral compounds that could be integrated into existing post-exposure regimens of passive and active immunization (23, 24); and

— advancing wildlife rabies control through oral vaccination, continued development of novel vaccines, baits, and baiting strategies, and objective assessment and additional generation of cost-benefit analyses of such strategies (29).

Conclusions and recommendations. These are outlined below.

• Although rabies is not considered eradicable at the present time, control of the disease in urban areas worldwide is feasible, and would reduce human mortality due to rabies and significant morbidity and economic costs associated with administration of post-exposure prophylaxis.

• Control of rabies in these circumstances may be facilitated by the development of an oral bait vaccine (23) for dogs.

• Although both the public and governments are aware of the health risks of rabies, a cost analysis of rabies post-exposure prophylaxis in developing countries may stimulate greater efforts to control the disease in those countries (28).

• International efforts to ensure the quality of rabies vaccines should be strengthened, and manufacturers urged to replace reactogenic brain-derived vaccine with safer cell-culture derived vaccines, as recommended by the WHO Expert Committee on Biological Standardization (24).

- Recent discoveries of previously unknown bat reservoirs of rabies virus underscore the importance of continued research to define the natural history of the disease (*30, 31*).

Japanese encephalitis

Japanese encephalitis cannot be eradicated because it is transmitted from natural reservoirs, but it can be controlled or eliminated with effective vaccines (*32, 33*). Neglected in discussions of diseases of international importance, Japanese encephalitis has a significant regional public health impact in Asia, where its high mortality rate and the large proportion of surviving children with permanent neurological sequelae contribute to a considerable disease burden (*34*). In the past several decades, the disease has spread to previously unaffected areas in Asia, as well as to territories in Australia and the Pacific (*35*).

Essential facilitating factors. An effective vaccine for Japanese encephalitis exists, and universal childhood immunization has led to the near elimination of the disease in Japan, Republic of Korea, and China (Province of Taiwan), where previously thousands of cases were reported annually (*33*). A significant regional reduction in disease incidence has been noted in areas of Thailand where the vaccine has been incorporated into EPI programmes (*34*). Interruption of viral transmission in the animal reservoirs, by vaccinating or removing pigs or by vector control, is an adjunct strategy, but cannot be solely relied upon to control the disease (*36*).

Essential impeding factors. While the current vaccine, which is derived from infected mouse brain, is effective, it requires two doses for primary immunization and numerous booster doses to maintain immunity (*33, 37*). The vaccine causes hypersensitivity reactions in 0.5% of those who receive it (*37, 38*). Vaccine production, supply, and cost are limited by the technical complexity of the manufacturing process. For many developing countries, lack of resources limits its use, despite political will to implement the vaccine into national programmes.

An alternative, live attenuated vaccine, produced and distributed in China, is safe and effective and has been used in more than 100 million children (*39*). Despite requiring two doses, the vaccine could be available at a lower cost than the current vaccine; however, it is currently licensed only in China.

Key strategies. The key to controlling Japanese encephalitis is to incorporate the vaccine into EPI programmes in Asia, This strategy has already been

shown to control the disease to the point of elimination in several countries.

Research needs. The priority for research is to develop an improved vaccine to replace the current inactivated vaccine. The live-attenuated vaccine available in China may fulfil some of the requirements, but there are uncertainties about its cost when produced under internationally accepted standards, and unresolved practical issues, such as its thermal stability, concurrent administration with other vaccines, and safety in HIV-infected children.

Conclusions and recommendations. These are shown below.

- Japanese encephalitis produces a significant burden of disease regionally in Asia, which can be prevented by routine childhood immunization.

- Control of the disease to the point of elimination has been demonstrated in several countries, and regional control is within reach with outside support of national programmes or by the development and use of a less expensive vaccine.

- With the emergence of the disease in new areas during recent decades, consideration should be given to more extensive control on a national and regional basis.

Acknowledgements

Thanks are due to Dr Hal Margolis, Dr Olen Kew, Dr J.M. Olivé, Dr Theodore Tsai, Dr Fred Robbins, Dr Luis Barreto, Dr Natth Bhamarapravati, and Dr Jaime Sepulveda for their special contributions to this report.

References

1. **Hadler SC.** Global impact of hepatitis A virus infection changing patterns. In: Hollinger FB et al. eds. *Viral hepatitis and liver disease.* Baltimore, MD, Williams & Wilkins, 1991: 14–20.
2. **Centers for Disease Control and Prevention.** Prevention of hepatitis A through active or passive immunization. Recommendations of the Advisory Committee on Immunization Practices. *Morbidity and mortality weekly report*, 1996, **45** (RR-15): 1–30.
3. **Shapiro CN, Margolis HS.** Worldwide epidemiology of hepatitis A virus infection. *Journal of hepatology*, 1994, **18** (suppl. 2): s11–14.
4. **Lemon SM.** Type A viral hepatitis: new developments in an old disease. *New England journal of medicine*, 1985, **313**: 1059–1067.
5. **Innis BL et al.** Protection against hepatitis A by an inactivated vaccine. *Journal of the American Medical Association*, 1994, **271**: 1328–1334.

6. **Werzberger A et al.** A controlled trial of formalin-inactivated hepatitis A vaccine in healthy children. *New England journal of medicine*, 1992, **327**: 453–457.

7. **Maynard JE, Kane MA, Hadler SC.** Global control of hepatitis B through vaccination: role of hepatitis B vaccine in the Expanded Programme on Immunization. *Reviews of infectious diseases*, 1989, **11**: s574–578.

8. **Olivé JM, Aylward BR, Melgaard B.** Disease eradication as a public health strategy: is measles next? *World health statistic quarterly*, 1997, **50**: 185–187.

9. **Murray CJL, Lopez AD,** eds. *The global burden of disease: a comprehensive assessment of mortality and disability from diseases, injuries, and risk factors in 1990 projected to 2020 — summary.* Geneva, World Health Organization, 1996: 17–26.

10. **Cutts FT.** *The immunological basis for immunization: measles.* Unpublished document WHO/EPI/GEN/93.17, 1993 (available upon request from Global Programme for Vaccines and Immunization, World Health Organization, 1211 Geneva 27, Switzerland).

11. **Expanded Programme on Immunization.** *EPI Information System: global summary, August 1997.* Unpublished document WHO/EPI/GEN 97.02 (available upon request from Global Programme for Vaccines and Immunization, World Health Organization, 1211 Geneva 27, Switzerland).

12. **Cutts FT et al.** Control of rubella and congenital rubella syndrome (CRS) in developing countries. 1: Burden of disease from CRS. *Bulletin of the World Health Organization*, 1997, **75**: 55–68.

13. **Robertson SE et al.** Control of rubella and congenital rubella syndrome (CRS) in developing countries. 2: Vaccination against rubella. *Bulletin of the World Health Organization*, 1997, **75**: 69–80.

14. **Monath TP.** Yellow fever: *Victor, victoria?* Conqueror, conquest? Epidemics and research in the last 40 years and prospects for the future. *American journal of tropical medicine and hygiene*, 1991, **45**: 1–43.

15. **Monath TP.** Yellow fever vaccine. In: Plotkin SA, Mortimer EA. eds. *Vaccines*, 3rd ed. Philadelphia, WB Saunders, (in press).

16. **Monath TP.** Epidemiology of yellow fever: current status and speculations on future trends. In: Saluzzo JF, Dodets G. eds. *Factors in the emergence of arbovirus diseases*. Paris, Elsevier, 1997: 143–156.

17. **Pan American Health Organization.** Present status of yellow fever: Memorandum from a PAHO meeting. *Bulletin of the World Health Organization*, 1986, **64**: 511–524.

18. **Gratz NA, Knudsen AB.** *The rise and spread of dengue, dengue haemorrhagic fever and its vectors — a historical review.* Unpublished document CTD/FIL (DEN) 96.7, 1996.

19. **Robertson SE et al.** Yellow fever: a decade of reemergence. *Journal of the American Medical Association*, 1996, **276**: 1157–1162.

20. *Prevention and control of yellow fever in Africa.* Geneva, World Health Organization, 1986.

21. **Monath TP, Nasidi A.** Should yellow fever vaccine be included in the Expanded Programme of Immunization in Africa? A cost-effectiveness analysis. *American journal of tropical medicine and hygiene*, 1993, **48**: 274–299.

22. **Centers for Disease Control and Prevention.** Compendium of animal rabies control, 1997. National Association of State Public Health Veterinarians, Inc. *Morbidity and mortality weekly report*, 1997, **46**: 1–9.

23. **Centers for Disease Control and Prevention.** Rabies prevention — United States, 1991: recommendations of the Immunization Practices Advisory Committee (ACIP). *Morbidity and mortality weekly report*, 1991, **40** (RR-3): 1–19.

24. *WHO Expert Committee on Rabies. Eighth Report.* Geneva, World Health Organization, 1992 (WHO Technical Report Series, No. 824).

25. *World survey of rabies No. 30 for the year 1994.* Unpublished WHO document WHO/EMC/ZOO/96.3, 1996.

26. **Baer GM.** Oral rabies vaccination: an overview. *Reviews of infectious diseases*, 1988, **10** (Suppl. 4): S644–S648.

27. **Smith JS, Orciari LA, Yager PA.** Molecular epidemiology of rabies in the United States. *Seminars in virology*, 1995, **6**: 387–400.

28. **Meslin F-X, Fishbein DB, Matter HC.** Rationale and prospects for rabies elimination in developing countries. In: Rupprecht CE et al. eds. *Current topics in microbiology and immunology*, Berlin, Springer-Verlag, 1994: 1–26.

29. **Rupprecht CE et al.** The ascension of wildlife rabies: a cause for public health concern or intervention? *Emerging infectious diseases*, 1995, **1**: 107–114.

30. **Hanlon CA, Rupprecht CE.** The reemergence of rabies. In: Scheld WM et al. eds. *Emerging infections*, Washington, DC, ASM Press: 1998: 59–80.

31. **Allworth A, Murray K, Morgan J.** A human case of encephalitis due to a lyssavirus recently identified in fruit bats. *Communicable diseases intelligence*, 1996, **20**: 504.

32. **Burke DS, Leake CJ.** Japanese encephalitis. In: Monath TP. ed. *The arboviruses: epidemiology and ecology*, Vol. III. Boca Raton, CRC Press, 1988: 63–92.

33. **Tsai TF, Chang GJ, Yu YX.** Japanese encephalitis vaccines. In: Plotkin S, Orenstein W. *Vaccines*, 3rd ed. Philadelphia, WB Saunders, (in press).

34. **Rojanosuphot S, Tsai TF.** eds. Regional workshop on control strategies for Japanese encephalitis. *Southeast Asia journal of tropical medicine and public Health*, 1995, **26** (S3): 1–59.

35. **Mackenzie JS et al.** Emergence of Japanese encephalitis virus in the Australasian region. In: Salluzzo JF, Dodet B. eds. *Factors in the emergence of arbovirus diseases*. Paris, Elsevier, 1997: 191–201.

36. **Vaughn DW, Hoke CH.** The epidemiology of Japanese encephalitis: prospects for prevention. *Epidemiological reviews*, 1992, **14**: 197–221.

37. **Centers for Disease Control and Prevention.** Inactivated Japanese encephalitis virus vaccine. Recommendations of the Advisory Committee on Immuni-

zation Practices (ACIP). *Morbidity and mortality weekly report*, 1993, **42** (RR-1).

38. **Plesner AM, Ronne T.** Allergic mucocutaneous reactions to Japanese encephalitis vaccine. *Vaccine*, 1997, **15**: 1239–1243.

39. **Hennessy S et al.** Effectiveness of live-attenuated Japanese encephalitis vaccine (SA14-14-2): a case–control study. *Lancet*, 1996, **347**: 1583–1586.

DISCUSSION AND SYNTHESIS

Comments and discussion following Workgroup Reports

Comment

In our Workgroup, as in a number of other groups, we had difficulty with the term "elimination" and discussed this at some length. Fortunately, we owe a great debt to the Dahlem Workshop in eradicating the phrase "elimination of a disease as a public health problem". A number of us would like to eradicate the word "elimination". I think control is a respectable term. I hope we would see ourselves as being sufficiently imaginative and creative to be able to frame progress in terms of control as being an exciting and saleable entity. If we are going to use "elimination", we need to use it as carefully as we use "eradication". It has to be a feasible goal, and we ought to be able to demonstrate that it is a feasible goal. I was a little concerned, particularly with the noninfectious disease group, when we talked about eliminating iron, iodine and vitamin A deficiencies and eliminating lead poisoning. I think we all have to agree that none of these are feasible goals. It would be helpful in their report if they were to redefine "elimination" as being low incidence; it is not a goal to eliminate these conditions. This only illustrates our problem with the word "elimination" and what we mean by it and what we are trying to mean by it. In our dictionary, "elimination" and "eradication" have identical meanings. In other languages, as I am told, it creates no end of confusion. There is no way of differentiating between the two.

Question

I have a question that is related to terminology but is perhaps more practical, bearing on the next-to-last recommendation for measles. The point was that efforts to address measles should not jeopardize programmes or efforts to eradicate poliomyelitis. That is the general recommendation. I wondered whether the group had considered giving some concrete examples to show how embarking on a more ambitious measles programme would not interfere with or jeopardize poliomyelitis eradication efforts. I ask for examples because one of the benefits of this meeting has been the juxtaposition of thinking about synergies in sustainable health development and a variety of different elimination or eradication programmes. Can we hear some creative thinking about concrete ways, operationally and conceptually, and how these programmes would harmonize, synergize, or potentiate one another's efforts?

Answer

I see the theoretical concern. I can give no example where a measles elimination programme has adversely affected poliomyelitis. In fact, I think they are mutually complementary. That has been my experience in Mexico. What we learned in poliomyelitis is now being applied to measles but without undoing our efforts to continue with poliomyelitis. These are synergistic efforts.

Comment

I would like to address a point that was brought out by one workgroup about special situations or special circumstances that make eradication particularly difficult in certain countries. Guinea-worm and poliomyelitis eradication efforts demonstrate that successful eradication efforts can be carried out in spite of war and conflict. What characterizes these countries is that a number of prerequisites for eradication are not present. The strategies for these situations (often without governments and without resources) are different from the strategies we advocate in the majority of countries. My suggestion is that the conference recognizes that the eradication prerequisites for these countries are different, strategies must be different, and funding needs are different. Special financing mechanisms must be created for eradication efforts in these countries.

Comment

I should like to respond to the question of competition between the measles and poliomyelitis eradication initiatives. The key issue here is planning and resources. In a number of instances, the country or an organization wanted to have what we would categorize as a multi-entity campaign — the idea being that since the poliomyelitis campaigns were already being conducted, additional entities could simply be added. The need for additional health personnel, trained administrators, or trained vaccinators who know how to handle syringes and needles safely without transmitting bloodborne diseases was not considered. Programmes can work together, but the key issues are proper planning and proper resources. An area where different programmes can work well together is surveillance. We feel strongly that measles surveillance is needed to keep good poliomyelitis surveillance in place through the period of certification. Without enthusiasm, without a particular goal, surveillance tends to deteriorate over time. Poliomyelitis and measles eradication efforts can work very closely together, very cooperatively, so let's focus on making sure we have the resources to do it.

Comment

My comment is in relation to rubella vaccine and the inclusion of it in measles eradication. There was one bullet in the Workgroup Report that referred to vaccinating women of childbearing age with rubella vaccine to accelerate rubella elimination. There is a view that you need to include both men and women in relation to rubella vaccination if you really want to eliminate rubella. The rubella virus continues to circulate in the population, and some women who are pregnant may still be affected, and you may get cases of CRS.

Comment

The terms "eradication" and "elimination" have other problems that don't have to do with science, but have to do with communication. In my work with the spina bifida community, some people are vastly offended when I talk about elimination or eradication, because either they or their children have spina bifida, and they see this as in some way ending their lives. It is amazing that this hasn't been mentioned by the poliomyelitis and other communities, but it certainly has come out of the chronic disability communities in this country. This is another reason to think about terms like "complete prevention" or "80% control", rather than eradication and elimination.

Comment

My comment concerns a suggestion made in both Group 1 (disease elimination/eradication) and Group 3 (bacterial diseases). In Group 3, for example, one of their recommendations for each condition was that control be tightly related to general health-delivery systems or sustainable health development. We're all talking about sustainable health development. The phrase "general health-delivery systems" is a little passive. It suggests that people are being passive beneficiaries in the transfer of resources and efforts. These statements should be strengthened to recognize that probably many of our efforts in control and eradication would be of lower cost and more effective if we were able to work with communities that are more aggressive in demanding health care and that are able to recognize their rights

to good health care. These diseases ought not to exist in communities that are well structured, well organized, and well mobilized. Community mobilization and organization in some peoples' terminology is part of sustainable health development and part of health-delivery systems, but I fear in some people's terminology, it isn't. I would like to strengthen the role of community participation.

Comment

I represent the Dutch government and I have to advise my government where to put our money. At this conference we have seen fantastic presentations, a contest of all the diseases we want to eradicate. We need financing for that. What is not clear from this conference is where do we put our money. I would like to compare certain diseases, certain interventions with others. Resources are limited — not only limited financially, but also limited in human capital. I would like to see cost-effectiveness data for these diseases. Which of the interventions is most cost-effective? We have a universal unit of measurement, the DALY, although it has many critics. One of the problems with DALYs is that they do not exactly apply to what we want here because of the need to include transmission. The only disease that is included is tuberculosis. We're definitely looking at what is the effect of intervention on the cost-effectiveness ratio. That's one of the good examples. The whole global burden of disease studies and cost-effectiveness for many other diseases is not clear at all. My recommendation is to look into these issues more specifically so we could compare one intervention with the other.

Comment

As a number of speakers have already expressed, there is a concern that as we go from eradication to elimination to control, this list has become very, very long and somewhat cumbersome and has now become the battle of diseases as just described. One of the things we have failed to do in this meeting is to discuss any approaches to prioritization. There is a science to this. It is well described in the literature. There are approaches to public health problem prioritization that lend themselves to some of this discussion. We haven't had time in any of the groups to really focus on it. Another way to look at this issue is to take examples of poliomyelitis and guinea-worm disease and ask why they are currently at the top of the list. What is the logical framework that has led them to move to that level in contrast to some of the other issues? Of the issues that we've talked about, certainly feasibility and effectiveness are the two major parameters. There may be others, but those certainly are the most important. If you constructed a 2×2 table, those things that ended up in cell A — highly feasible with a highly effective intervention available — would be very top candidates for elimination. This would maybe address the concern about where to put the money. We need to be clear about describing what we mean by effectiveness. Much of the debate of the disease groups has focused on the question of efficacy, in addition to acceptability. Those two combined add up to effectiveness. The classic example of that is that you can use efficacious interventions such as condoms for HIV; and if it is unacceptable, you don't have a very effective intervention.

Feasibility is much more difficult to discuss. We've touched on some key issues of this, not the least of which is infrastructure concerns. Some of the groups tried to deal with that — infrastructure concerns for both the service delivery, the ability to deliver whatever the intervention is, and surveillance to detect and monitor. Those two key factors are extremely important.

Resource constraints: we mentioned that, but if the resources are available and the political will is not there, that is a major consideration. What factors affect political will? Certainly the size of the problem in terms of prevalence, but also severe DALY measures, case-fatality rates, and other issues.

And last but not least, urgency. We've heard that issue come up again and again, which includes economic impact, infectious spread, and other issues that relate to that. So those are just some of the issues we can begin to discuss at some point. Perhaps not at this meeting, but in future ones. How to prioritize these? How to figure the appropriate weights of those elements? Where is the sensitivity analysis to guide where to put our emphasis? These might help us prioritize this very lengthy list of diseases and steer us in some of the right directions to help us spend our resources, time, and energy wisely.

Comment

My major concern is what will be next after this conference. I see that Dr Foege, after the break, will talk about "Vision for the future." But we have a very short list of diseases that are eradicable or can be eliminated. Probably this short list is a reflection more of our ignorance at the present time than actually the limits of science and technology and whatever the people can do. And I would like to recommend two things: that as an outcome of the conference, we actually make a proposal, and each organization and all the people involved are to allocate more resources in terms of research, including

operational research (i.e. how to involve the communities) so we can actually move forward.

The second proposal I would like to make is that we bring the recommendations of this conference to other forums, particularly public health forums, so that efforts we have made can be put into action.

Comment

I'm really picking up some of the comments from the last couple of speakers. We don't have a lot of time and ability to try to refine further the work that has been done by the workgroups who have done enormous amounts under enormous pressure. Further work needs to be done, and I hope the conference is going to be giving a fairly broad mandate to the further editorial work of sifting down and clarifying, where we can, what seems to be a consensus. I think that the report should be as clear as it can in whatever can be distilled from what we said.

I certainly agree that we should do better with our priorities, better with our analysis, and better with our DALYs, but international development still remains far more of an art than a science. I hate to say it to our colleagues who are having a terrible problem of allocating resources from international development agencies, but you are not going to get a menu that's going to solve your problems. It's going to remain extremely difficult, although we need to do a better job than we're doing now in helping that process. We have that same problem also in WHO.

The definition problem has been raised by many. I don't see exactly a consensus. I see uncomfortableness expressed with how our current usage goes, not total comfortableness with the Dahlem recommendations. I wonder if the conference organizers or the secretariat who will be working on this further might consider if they can distil what they really feel is consensus from the conference, or even convene a small informal working group and put this as an annex to the conference report which would say, "Look, this seems to us . . . " — because we are not ready to express the consensus of this conference, we haven't had the chance to endorse it. We need some further work so that we have something concrete to work on, so we can take that into other forums and see what to do with it. As I said, one way of doing this is to have a small working group and publish their report in an annex.

Other things about other forums: I hope my colleagues in WHO will work with me in trying to take some of the specific recommendations on tuberculosis and perhaps Chagas disease, certainly for the global programme on vaccines and immunizations on rubella and measles and feed those into our current expert advisory groups so we can look at them in more detail. Maybe they will give us some new insights; maybe there are ways that we can use those. Recommendations from those technical advisory groups can be published in the WHO *Weekly epidemiological record* and in other forums — and maybe in a World Health Assembly resolution. As you know, this conference report will be published as a special supplement to the *Bulletin of the World Health Organization*. So that is another way of bringing it into international visibility.

My last comment is about too many diseases being candidates for eradication. WHO should be doing a better job in its role as a gate-keeper. I can speak from my own experience: when one enthusiastic programme manager says, "Let's do this, let's go for an elimination programme. I've got some wonderful NGOs. They're enthusiastic. We've got resources, let's go for it," I say, "Sure, let's do it." But we have not yet had in WHO really an upper, senior level management where we can debate with all the programmes and say, "Okay, how many of these things should go to the World Health Assembly?" This is not something that I can do inside WHO. You who will be coming to our Executive Board and will be attending the World Health Assembly can help with that process.

Comment

Fundamental to what we're trying to do here is reaching agreement on the basic framework — that is, whether to include eradication, elimination, and control, or just eradication and control. It's very tempting for each of us to address that issue on the basis of political or personal commitment to our pet diseases, and there are obviously dangers involved in doing that. It makes much more sense for us to be asking a question of whether the strategies involved with control — e.g. for infectious diseases in hyperendemic phases, or even decline phases — are the same as the strategies that are necessary for elimination. And are those the same as strategies necessary for eradication? There is a growing volume of work in the literature, at least for infectious or communicable diseases, that say specific strategies or combinations of strategies do differ, and that we ought to be looking at this in a more sophisticated way. My personal bias is that the strategies do differ for at least the communicable diseases, and therefore it is important for us to agree on retaining elimination as a category.

Comment

Two comments and a question. First of all, much of this meeting has been talking about making possible

what to others would seem impossible, and accomplishing what many would say is impossible. And that is a wonderful setting for heroes and stories. Second, the future of health, the world, etc. is in the hands of our youth. The question: Are we doing enough in taking these stories and examples of heroes — many are in this room, and also the local community level — and using them to develop and grow the leaders of the future?

Comment

With regard to the price of some new products being a perceived barrier to their wider use, I would like to comment on the pricing of products and the value of prevention. DPT vaccines were licensed at least 25–50 years ago, and it took us a long time to get these into wide use. Smallpox vaccine took even longer. Those vaccines that are now used at prices well under US$ 1 a dose have come to that pricing because of economies of scale and the learning curve that was 25–50 years long. What we are trying to do now in many cases is put products into wide use much earlier in their life-cycle, without the benefit of experience in increasing the efficiency of production. If you do cost-effectiveness analysis on hepatitis B vaccine at under US$ 1 a dose, perhaps down to US$ 0.50, and hepatitis A vaccine at US$ 3 per dose or perhaps slightly less, these vaccines in many developing countries are still cost-saving. In poorer countries, where they spend less on treatment, they still buy a unit of health benefit, whether a life saved or a DALY saved, at a value that the World Bank represents as a very good investment.

Clearly, we need to try to make vaccines more affordable. To get the price down, we have to get the number of doses up, and we need to target external assistance to those countries that are most in need of it. But the reality is that prices in the manufacture of many new products will never fall to the level we currently experience for poliomyelitis or measles vaccines. So we have to address the reality that many new products in their early life-cycle will be more expensive. We have to convince governments that investing in the use of these vaccines, in investing in prevention, is a good health investment.

Dean Jamison said very early in the conference that there was increasing evidence that investing in health is good for the overall economy of the country. We have to get this message out. Advocacy for investing in health must be a much bigger part of the overall strategy. We must use more sophisticated techniques for advocacy and the decision-making process. Many scientific advances are accumulating at the moment, many new vaccines that are in the pipeline will be licensed in the next few years, and there are probably many other technologies for drugs. These new products are not going to get to most developing countries in an acceptable time frame. We need to regard advocacy and changing the behaviour of government resource providers as a very significant part of the overall health strategy.

Comment

One thing I was hoping to hear from the meeting is what is the overall goal of eradication/elimination. We need to revisit that. Lastly, let us remember that knowledge also comes through practice. It is sometimes disheartening if we think that knowledge only comes through science and do not remember that there are people out there who have knowledge gathered through practice which could be shared in terms of strategy development. Many people out there will spend a lot of their time working with communities and working in districts — developing strategies that could be part of this process of sharing.

Conference synthesis and vision for the future

W.H. Foege[1]

Eric Hofer once remarked, "When everything has already been said, be brief, repeat, exaggerate." I can't exaggerate about how good, how useful, how stimulating this meeting has been. Peter Drucker has said that everything must degenerate into work if anything is to happen. The amount of work done here in the last 52 hours predicts that much will happen in the future.

Last night, I gave a talk at Emory University entitled, "Protect the future, you may be living there." The two points that I hoped to make were, first, the immortality of all of our actions, and second, perspective. For perspective I started with a story: Abd-er-Rahman III (912–961 AD), a powerful ruler of a dynasty in Spain 1000 years ago, left behind a note at his death:

"I have now reigned above 50 years in victory or peace ... Riches and honors, powers and pleasures, have waited on my call; nor does any earthly blessing appear to have been wanting to my felicity. In this situation I have diligently numbered the days of pure and genuine happiness which have fallen to my lot. They amount to fourteen."

What a sad commentary. For immortality, I spent some time making the case that we are not just tied to the past, but we are tied to every detail of the past. Likewise, it is not just the general actions, but every detail of today that has implications for the future. That is where Rafe Henderson started on Monday morning. If we are to do good, it will be in the details.

Many people will spend today, as they spent yesterday, and everyday, with all of their talent and energies devoted to making money — trading stocks, trying to figure out how to sell more cigarettes, scheming to separate money from other people. Those actions are immortal with many ripples into the future ... but they aren't necessarily important. Richard Hamming has said, "If you want to do important work, you have to work on important problems." What you have done in the past 3 days, which is possible because of what you have done over the years, is important work. To this end, I offer the following observations.

Observation 1. A PROCESS HAS BEEN BORN. This process builds on Dahlem and many things preceding, but it now has a secure life of its own.

- You have pushed for some order, some priority, some balance in deciding the specific eradication targets that make sense.

- You have developed a road map for organizing people and resources in the future.

- But most important, you have catalysed a process for refining, making corrections and promoting these ideas in the future. This process is very similar to the 1990 objectives: they started in 1978 with a meeting in Atlanta; some 220 objectives were selected for 1990, many so bad that they could not even be measured in 1990. But by setting targets the critics were able to have specific things to attack which gave us a chance to improve the targets and the definitions.

What we learned from the 1990 objectives is the power of the process. We don't have to have all of the answers. We don't even have to have all of the definitions right. What we have is a process that, just like science itself, is self correcting and keeps improving on the answers. Healthy people 2000 will be better than the 1990 objectives and the 2010 objectives will be even better.

We have only 50 years of experience in global organizations, and only 30 years of experience with successful eradication programmes. It is no wonder that we are still struggling to find the best way to organize, to implement, to cooperate. But struggle we must, because we cannot afford to waste resources, or time, or effort when the problems require the best we have to offer collectively. Rafe is right: the organizers need to edit the results, provide their own conclusions and plan the next steps.

Observation 2. A FRESH LOOK. You have tried to take a fresh look at disease eradication and control. There is power in doing that as a way of life; some examples:

- People used to ask: Why is a mirror reversed from left to right but not top to bottom? Richard Feynman, the physicist, took a fresh look. He says it is psychological rather than real. It is front and back that are reversed, as if you were squashed

[1] Rollins School of Public Health, Emory University, Atlanta, GA, USA.

back to front. Since we cannot imagine that, we make it left to right.

- Another example. For centuries, people believed that Aristotle was right when he said that the heavier an object, the faster it would fall to earth. Aristotle was regarded as the greatest thinker of all times and surely he could not be wrong. All it would have taken was for one brave person to take two objects, one heavy and one light, and drop them from a great height to see whether or not the heavier object landed first. But no one stepped forward until nearly 2000 years after Aristotle's death. In 1589, Galileo summoned learned professors to the base of the Leaning Tower of Pisa. Then he went to the top and pushed off a ten-pound and a one-pound weight. Both landed at the same time. Case closed? No. The power of belief in the conventional wisdom was so strong that the professors denied what they had seen. They continued to say that Aristotle was right.

- A final example. In September 1942 a request was received from Guadalcanal for 100 gross of medical item #75–177, condoms. It made no sense; so the request went all the way up to Admiral Nimitz because no one could figure out why they would be wanted. He read the request and immediately said that General Vandegrift probably needs them to keep the rain out of the marines' rifles. He was right. Both of these leaders looked at things in a different way.

I have a hard time dropping beliefs just because they happen to be wrong. But here we have had the chance to revisit and test our beliefs, our approaches, our assumptions and our abilities. And we did. We pointed out where the survey was not helpful, and where definitions were confused. What would happen if we changed the question? What if we gave great rewards to the person who could develop a programme to save the world from the loss of 100 million DALYs each year? What would the programme look like: How much in control, how much in eradication? What is the maximum outcome we could buy for a billion dollars a year? How does that inform the debate about eradication and control?

Observation 3. DEFINITIONS. Bjorn Melgaard pointed out that it is not useful to polarize the debate. Some of you have heard me say that before speaking at the 1986 American Public Health Association meeting where I reviewed the materials from the programme 100 years earlier. To my great surprise, I found that public health people in this country were debating vertical versus horizontal programmes. I wondered if we were wasting time and

asked what had actually happened in the USA during those 100 years. The answer won't surprise you. We actually implemented things whenever we had the tools, often in very vertical ways, with the result that we kept enlarging the infrastructure which was able to constantly take on new challenges.

The CDC infrastructure was forged from work on a single disease. In the early 1940s, the first task of what would become CDC was to provide a 1-mile mosquito-free barrier around every military installation in the south so that recruits being trained for the Second World War would not get malaria. After the war, with the addition of each new vertical programme, the general capacity for public health developed. But even now, CDC has trouble getting appropriations for infrastructure. Congress wants to fund AIDS or diabetes or immunization programmes. The challenge for CDC leadership is to see a big picture and then capitalize on the individual skills and interests of its employees and the single-issue fanaticism of its funders. I have frequently said that we have to tie the needs of the poor to the fears of the rich if we are to get anyplace.

The bottom line? As eradication efforts improve the credibility, power, and attention to public health, the infrastructure improves. As the infrastructure improves we have greater opportunities, skills and tools to consider eradication. The mix is so important that we must beware of using words that may divide our effort. Kipling said that "Words are the most powerful drug in the world." We must use words with care, to bind and promote public health rather than to divide our efforts. Petrarch, the father of the Renaissance, distrusted philosophers because he said they became too clever with words — great debaters, but hardly wise. We want to be wise rather than great debaters. Unifiers, healers. To be wise, let's use the words as now defined, but challenge everyone to come up with better ideas on a continuing basis. As Don Hopkins suggested, don't cheapen the word eradication when you mean control.

And we need to figure out how to communicate to others. Godfrey Oakley mentioned one difficulty this morning with the terms eradication and elimination. On Sunday, I talked to a politician, very influential in the funding of public health programmes in this country. I talked about DALYs and return on investment and the need to tie resources to the size of the health problem. Basically, the politician's message was: this will not work; you must go back to the drawing board if you want to have an impact on politicians; get us emotionally involved in specifics; and target your efforts.

As we debated definitions I found myself thinking about our efforts over the years to attack measles in the USA. The problem was to avoid an objective that would cause us to stop short of what was actually possible. I recall the pleas not to choose interruption of transmission as a goal because if we failed, that would certainly set back public health. But we knew that anything less would not reveal the ultimate barriers. We set the objective of interrupting indigenous transmission and we reviewed our efforts once a week. It was indeed like peeling an onion and finding new layers of problems: school outbreaks led to changes in school entry requirements; measles in military recruits caused the military to change procedures; measles in day-care centres prompted entry requirements; and different solutions were required for other situations, including special groups, such as drum and bugle corps members, and wrestlers, college students, and people attending social functions such as weddings. Each new problem required a new solution. But without the goal of interrupting transmission, that would not have been found. Finally we came to the ultimate barrier . . . importation, forcing us to look at the global picture. My point is, we must balance a line of not raising expectations by using the wrong words, but not settle for anything short of what might actually be possible.

Observation 4. This follows from the preceding observation. Rick Goodman raised the question of "synergy". It may be hard to measure, but it is a message I get from this discussion. Denis Broun pointed out the tension between eradication and other things. Of course, it is the balancing of tension that produces new molecules, compounds and products. For example, many speakers mentioned the key ingredients required for both eradication and infrastructure: surveillance, epidemiology, analysis, implementation, logistics, evaluation, etc. These ingredients are not only necessary for both, but are refined in different ways by both and then reinforce each other.

We heard convincing evidence that **eradication contributes to infrastructure.** This contribution is reflected through factors, including political involvement, the power of success, techniques and tools, and mobilization of resources, as shown by the role of Rotary International in poliomyelitis eradication. This effort brings new money for health programmes, not a diversion of health money. Don Hopkins pointed out that guinea-worm eradication is taking primary health care to places that never had it before. What are the other possibilities? What does the Rotary involvement teach us about broadening our base of public support?

It made me think back to several years ago in the Congo when I visited a health centre without prior notice. On the wall they had an impressive chart showing immunization status. I asked them how they checked to make sure it was really that good. They said, "We use the Henderson method." I said, "Tell me about that." They then described the 30-cluster technique that we all know. The Henderson method was developed 30 years ago when Rafe Henderson was conducting an evaluation of the smallpox programme in West Africa. He enlisted the help of Don Eddins who used techniques developed by Sherman and Serfling in the USA and figured out how to make them applicable to a developing country. So the infrastructure of U.S. public health provided techniques for an eradication programme which in turn have become part of the infrastructure of primary health care. *There in one story is the lesson we should be taking away*.

There are other lessons. Eradication contributed to the progress of surveillance — the ease of use of the concept; since smallpox eradication, surveillance is used with a familiarity that wasn't possible before — to the CDC/WHO relationship, a relationship that was forged in the smallpox eradication campaign but is now part of the infrastructure; to laboratory techniques, upgrading, and standards, and to standardization of vaccines.

Another lesson. **infrastructure contributes to eradication.** The components of the system — vaccinators, health education, logistics, etc. — were invaluable to the smallpox campaign. Experiences in surveillance help us define the problem, define the possible, find the truth, the real, and the authentic. (I sometimes think of a true story of a man taking a picture at the wax museum in Washington, DC. He asked a woman with two grandchildren if they would kindly move for him to get a picture of the wax dummy of Lady Bird Johnson. He never realized that he asked Lady Bird Johnson and her two granddaughters to move so he could get a picture of a wax figure.) Infrastructure also contributes to evaluation and logistics systems. Indeed, every experience we have ever had in public health becomes part of the response we can muster for eradication.

Observation 5. MAKING THE CASE. I believe the burden lies with those interested in eradication to make a very persuasive case. Accept a high burden of proof that includes the points below.

- Make the case for reductions in suffering and death in individual countries and in the world. To be worth the effort of eradication, the problem to be solved must be significant.

- There must be an adequate return on investment as compared to other investments in health activities. Eradication does not get special consideration unless you can show a return on investment by DALYs or other similar measures.

- Demonstrate the benefits in terms of development. Those engaged in development activities tend to devalue the importance of health. We must be careful not to do the same thing in reverse. It is important to show that disease eradication is an important ingredient in improving development.

- Demonstrate the benefits in terms of strengthening the health infrastructure. As already stated, I believe the way to strengthen infrastructure is by solving health problems. But we need to be explicit. We need strategies that make it clear that infrastructure is being helped.

- Understand the risks incurred. And show that the benefits make this risk-taking appropriate (we took risks giving smallpox vaccine but we tried to calculate them). Think it through. Know the downside. Know it better than anyone who is trying to argue against the programme.

- Demonstrate in a geographical area, as D.A. Henderson was emphasizing, that it is possible. Again, there is a delicate balance. We must be able to see what is possible to believe. On the other hand, we have to believe some things if they are to be seen. There is no question that some risk-taking is required.

In summary, know the problems: acknowledge the real and potential problems of eradication, including the diversion of resources. Make the case for each eradication proposal with real care: What is the return on investment? What are the returns in terms of development? What are the returns in terms of stronger infrastructure?

We need better ways of calculating the value. Discounting may be fair in figuring the value of money now as compared to the future, but the bottom line is that it gives a different value to future people. Public health teaches us that the value of a person in Burundi is the same as one in Atlanta. That concept of social justice should place the same value on a person born next year or in 10 years or in 50 years. How do we avoid discounting the value of people?

I should add that public health does not always value economists appropriately. We quote Ezra Solomon, the economist; "The only function of economic forecasting is to make astrology look respectable." The fact is, just as lawyers have done a better job on tobacco than public health people, so have economists developed metrics for measuring the burden of disease that we were not able to develop on our own. I especially appreciated Dean Jamison's observation that the war on poverty may be through public health.

When we have done all of these things, and when the case is convincing, we must — yes, must —

then proceed to eradication of guinea-worm disease and poliomyelitis with conviction, with energy, with purpose, with leadership, and with a shared vision — as we did with samllpox. Because the benefits are impressive, some things need be done but once in the history of the world. Therefore, eradication is the ultimate in sustainability. Long term, it is also the ultimate in efficiency . . . and long term is the way that public health people should think. Eradication then, at its best, becomes a tugboat to pull other health programmes — it energizes health workers and builds social capital and social efficacy.

But the bottom line is that eradication attacks inequities and provides the ultimate in social justice. We say that is the base of public health philosophy, but only once has it been achieved in public health. In the last 20 years there has not been one case of smallpox because everyone in the world, and all of those yet to come, benefit from the experience and the knowledge acquired about that particular disease problem. Some make the argument that we have no right to impose poliomyelitis eradication on Africa. I understand that concern, but I am plagued by the opposite. Gandhi said his idea of the golden rule was that he couldn't have what was denied to others. If my children are protected from poliomyelitis I feel an obligation to share that with other parents. As Primo Levi has said, when we know how to prevent torment and don't, then we become the tormentors.

So the hurdle is high. We must meet high standards for eradication. But when these conditions are met, then we should make no mistake . . . eradication is the thing to pursue. Norman Cousins in a 1976 editorial asked what is the major gift that the United States has given the world. His answer was that the major gift has been that it is possible to plan a rational future. The Constitution is the incarnation of that idea. We fully believe it is not only possible, but mandatory, to plan a rational *health* future. We will be judged by how well we do for those separated by both geography and time. It is a challenge and a responsibility to "harmonize the trumpets".

Finally, to return to the idea of immortality. Abraham Lincoln, 133 years after his death, has left no biological DNA evidence that he lived. But every day we are influenced by the fact that he was here. He has left the social equivalent of DNA. The future may have your DNA, if telomerase works, or it may have parts of your DNA in your descendants, but it will for sure contain the fingerprints of your social DNA, the impact of all the decisions you make and the actions you take, the details accomplished. Your immortality is assured. Thanks for being part of this immortal work.

Post-conference Small Group report*

Below is presented a summary of the discussions of the Small Group which convened in Atlanta on 1–2 June 1998.

Definitions

Disease "elimination" (connoting something less than global implementation and requiring continued control measures) and "eradication" (connoting global implementation with no need for continuing control measures) have been in use for many years and have become common and useful terms to many public health practitioners. In 1997 the Dahlem Workshop added further legitimacy to these terms. However, discussions at the Conference on Global Disease Elimination and Eradication as Public Health Strategies confirmed the feelings of many that the distinction between elimination and eradication is difficult to convey. The two terms are synonymous in many languages. Adding to the confusion is the imaginative, but imprecise, use of the term elimination as, for example, in "elimination of the disease as a public health problem". The group reviewed the concerns expressed at the Conference and concluded that discontinuation of the term "elimination" be considered, using instead degrees of control leading, where feasible, to eradication. For example:

Control: The reduction of disease in a defined geographical area as a result of deliberate efforts. Control is a relative term that should be quantified to indicate the extent of reduction to be achieved.

Eradication: The absence of a disease agent in nature in a defined geographical area as the result of deliberate control efforts. Control measures can be discontinued when the risk of disease importation is no longer present.

Extinction: The specific disease agent no longer exists in nature or the laboratory.

* Members of the small group, listed in alphabetical order, were Stephen Cochi, Ciro de Quadros, Walter Dowdle, Richard Goodman, Peter Ndumbe, David Salisbury, Roland Sutter, and Frederick Trowbridge.

In effect, the term elimination is replaced by the concept of "regional eradication". The group recognizes that the sentiment expressed at the Conference to revise the definitions comes only a year after endorsement and refinement of the terms at the Dahlem Workshop, where it was suggested that the term regional eradication is contradictory. The debate is unlikely to end here. Words are defined by common usage. The simplified definitions are proposed to reduce misunderstanding and confusion among the intended audience and wider discussion of these definitions in other forums is urged.

Next steps

Based on suggestions offered during the Conference, the group proposes the following next steps:

• National governments, WHO, and other international agencies should adopt the principles outlined in this report for planning disease control and eradication activities.

• New disease control and eradication initiatives should involve the widest possible consultation to ensure that all opportunities are taken to maximize health gains.

• The Conference Proceedings published as a Supplement to the *Bulletin of the World Health Organization* should be broadly disseminated to ministries of health, key groups and organizations, and international health agencies.

• The *Summary* and the *Post-conference Small Group report* should be submitted to appropriate public health and policy journals and key individuals and organizations and placed on the WHO website.

• Discussion of this report should be included in meetings that address single disease initiatives to emphasize the opportunities for complementarity when control and eradication efforts for multiple diseases are implemented simultaneously.

• A follow-up international meeting should be convened in the year 2001 to review progress and consider new goals in disease control and eradication.

Annex A

FACT SHEETS FOR CANDIDATE DISEASES FOR ELIMINATION OR ERADICATION

1. Noninfectious conditions

Folic-acid-preventable spina bifida and anencephaly*

1. Brief description of the condition/disease

Spina bifida and anencephaly are among the most common and severe birth defects. Almost all affected persons with spina bifida have lower-body paralysis and significant physical disability. In many countries spina bifida is the most common cause of infantile paralysis. Anencephaly is a common birth defect that contributes to fetal and infant mortality.

An estimated 50–75% of these birth defects can be prevented by providing adequate intakes of synthetic folic acid (pteroylmonoglutamic acid) before and during the first trimester of pregnancy. Preventing folic-acid-preventable spina bifida and anencephaly presents an outstanding opportunity to improve the health of children throughout the world. Moreover, substantial evidence suggests that, in adults, suboptimal intake of folic acid is a major factor for increasing the risk of cardiovascular disease.

2. Current burden and rating within the overall burden of disease

Each year, 300 000 to 400 000 infants worldwide are born with spina bifida and anencephaly. In China, 100 000 infants are born annually with these two birth defects, which are the leading cause of infant mortality. The rates are also high in Mexico and Central America. Together these conditions contribute significantly to infant morbidity and mortality.

3. Feasibility (biological) of elimination/eradication

Approximately 75% of spina bifida and anencephaly are folic-acid-preventable, and it is biologically possible to prevent *all* folic-acid-preventable spina

bifida and anencephaly. The prevention impact would be approximately equal to the prevention derived from poliomyelitis vaccines.

The biological feasibility of preventing spina bifida and anencephaly using folic acid-containing vitamin supplements has been demonstrated in randomized controlled trials and other studies. Data from these studies indicate a 50–100% reduction in risk for women taking the supplement before conception and during the first trimester of pregnancy. No randomized controlled studies indicate that dietary changes alone will prevent these birth defects.

The U.S. Public Health Service recommends that all women who could become pregnant should consume 400μg of folic acid daily to prevent these birth defects. Many other countries have policy statements seeking to increase consumption. The United States Institute of Medicine recommended in April 1998 that all women who could become pregnant should consume 400μg daily of synthetic folic acid to prevent birth defects.

4. Estimated costs and benefits of elimination/eradication

Folic acid fortification of flour is feasible and inexpensive. In the USA, formal analysis of costs and benefits of fortification of wheat flour and other grains indicate that a fortification strategy would be highly cost-beneficial. Because costs associated with the purchase and distribution of folic-acid-containing supplements would be higher, programmes depending on pill consumption would break even.

5. Key strategies to accomplish the objectives

Folic acid intake to prevent folic-acid-preventable spina bifida and anencephaly can be increased by fortifying staple foods with folic acid or implementing a programme that increases the consumption of

* Contributed by Godfrey P. Oakley, Jr, Centers for Disease Control and Prevention, Atlanta, GA, USA.

folic-acid-containing supplements, as follows: fortify with synthetic folic acid one or more centrally processed and distributed foods, such as grain products, so that the vast majority of reproductive-aged women consume at least 400µg of folic acid each day; establish folic acid vitamin pill consumption programmes; add folic acid to iron supplement pill programs; and add folic acid to contraceptive pills.

6. Research needs

Cost-effective methods for population assessment of blood folate levels need to be field tested and improved. Such indicators of folate status are needed to provide a reliable means of evaluating the effectiveness of folic acid intervention programmes. Research is needed to develop messages that will motivate women to consume more folic acid.

7. Status of elimination/eradication efforts to date

Although many countries have developed recommendations to increase the consumption of folic acid, more needs to be done to implement these strategies. In the USA, 3 of 4 reproductive-aged women have blood folate levels that place them at risk of having a child with a folic-acid-preventable birth defect. Data from Europe are similar. The USA and China are implementing programmes to increase folic acid intakes. Approximately 20 other countries encourage the use of folic-acid-containing vitamins and the consumption of folate-rich foods. The USA and a few other countries have fortified one or more grain products with folic acid. Fortification concentration levels, however, so far have not been sufficient for complete prevention of these preventable birth defects.

8. Principal challenges to elimination/eradication

The principal challenges to eliminating folic-acid-preventable birth defects are a lack of awareness of this prevention opportunity by health care providers, policy-makers, and the public; the financial burden and logistical barriers to providing supplements to women; lack of centrally processed and distributed foods to serve as fortification vehicles in some countries; regulations in some countries limiting the amount of folic acid in supplement pills; misinterpretation of data, resulting in recommendation to promote only increased consumption of folate-rich foods rather than an adequate fortification or supplement programme with crystalline folic acid (pteroylmonoglutamic acid); and unwillingness of government to set fortification concentration levels high enough.

Iodine deficiency*

1. Brief description of the condition/disease

Iodine deficiency disorders (IDD) result from insufficient iodine in the environment and inadequate intake of iodine from food. Because development of the central nervous system depends on an adequate supply of thyroid hormone, which requires iodine for biosynthesis, iodine is an essential micronutrient for normal intellectual development and function. Endemic cretinism is the most severe manifestation of the lack of maternal and fetal thyroid hormone caused by severe dietary iodine deficiency; community-based assessments and iodine intervention trials indicate that IDD can leave entire populations with reduced intellectual capacity and impaired motor functions. Mild iodine deficiency can reduce the average population cognitive scores by 10–15%. Goitre, the most obvious clinical manifestation, frequently occurs in iodine-deficient populations.

2. Current global burden and ranking within the overall burden of disease

In 1991, using the most current data, WHO estimated that 20% of people throughout the world lived in areas in which iodine intake was inadequate. Subsequently, data became available that showed major cities in most of the developing world were also affected. In one study, 30–80% of neonates living in Asian cities had elevated TSH levels (>5 mU/l), indicating lack of iodine during the critical phase of brain development. The WHO estimates excluded data from states in the former Soviet Union, where iodized salt is generally unavailable, and where it is now known that the entire population lacks adequate iodine intake.

Since 1990, worldwide production and availability of iodized salt has increased greatly; production of iodized salt has increased from $<10\%$ to $>50\%$ in south-east Asia and India, $>70\%$ in China and Africa, and $>80\%$ in Latin America. Questions about iodized salt were included in the UNICEF-supported, household surveys conducted in 1996 in 50 countries; these surveys indicate that in 27 developing countries $>90\%$ of households use iodized salt, and in 15 countries 75–90% of households use iodized salt. In 1994, a total of 48 developing countries with IDD had no significant salt-iodization programmes; today, most of them have iodized more than half their salt. However, because problems with obtaining and maintaining the optimum level of iodine in salt have been widespread in most countries, iodine levels often are inadequate or, occasionally, too high to afford the best protection.

The global burden of disease (Christopher Murray & Alan Lopez, editors) ranked iodine deficiency in 1990 at 77, with 1562000 disability-adjusted life years (DALY); this estimate was based on the 1990 WHO data, which focused on the severe clinical manifestations of iodine deficiency and did not estimate the more widespread impact of reduced intellectual capacity in entire populations. With the success of salt iodization in most countries, the global burden of IDD has greatly decreased. However, further efforts are needed in many countries, and programmes must be maintained if IDD is to be permanently controlled.

3. Feasibility (biological) of elimination/eradication

Using salt iodization, it is possible to eliminate iodine deficiency as a public health problem and to employ sensitive biological markers to document this success. The principal challenge to elimination is the permanent intervention of adequate dietary iodine intake. In both developed and developing countries, iodine deficiency was eliminated, then recurred because of a lack of vigilance and a breakdown in the continuation of the intervention. Permanent elimination of iodine deficiency requires collaboration among private salt producers and government sectors to promote and monitor the use of iodized salt or other iodine-containing foods.

4. Estimated costs and benefits of elimination/eradication

Few estimates have been published of the costs and benefits. In 1993, the World Bank estimated an attractive US$ 8 DALY cost for iodine elimination through salt fortification. The estimated cost in India in 1994 was US$ 0.02–0.05 per person per year. The cost of salt fortification depends on the type of salt

---

* Contributed by Glen Maberly, Rollins School of Public Health, Emory University, Atlanta, GA, USA.

fortified and current practices; in areas with large manufacturers producing high-quality salt, the cost to iodize is <5% of production. The greatest cost is in packaging and labelling. If the salt is already packaged and labelled, the costs are insignificant. If the entire process is upgraded, as in China (representing about one-third of the global population), the investment is approximately US$ 100 million. In 1991, UNICEF estimated that US$ 100 million (in addition to the expected investments from national governments and local industry) would be necessary to achieve the mid-decade goal of Universal Salt Iodization. From 1993 through mid-1997, bilateral, multilateral development agencies and Kiwanis have invested approximately US$ 60 million for IDD elimination. Continued investments are necessary to ensure success and sustainability of IDD elimination.

5. Key strategies to accomplish the objective

Critical to any national IDD elimination programme requiring salt iodization are policies, laws, and agreements requiring all edible salt to be iodized, effective inspection and enforcement systems, and political advocacy and scientific support from community leaders. Ultimately, consumers need to be aware of the benefits so that the less expensive, unauthorized, noniodized salt does not persist in the market. Inclusion of salt testing and community education through school programmes has been effective in many countries. Because most salt is now produced by large-scale producers, once iodization is adopted and the best manufacturing practices are implemented, the impact can be massive and quality-control maintained. Salt iodization has been most difficult to implement and control in the tens of thousands of small-scale, cottage-industry producers.

Quality control in salt production and iodization is not common practice and is one of the greatest challenges to eliminating IDD. Simply providing salt iodization equipment is not the long-term answer. The development of cooperatives for iodization and use of micro-credit systems have been successful in some cases. Because establishing and maintaining laboratories capable of quality assurance of salt and measuring biological indicators have not been a priority for governments or agencies, long-term facilities for monitoring elimination and ensuring surveillance are widely lacking. Despite substantial achievements towards IDD elimination, the magnitude of iodine deficiency, its devastating impact on intellectual capacity, and the cost-benefit of its elimination are generally not well known beyond a small

group of development professionals. Overcoming this communication deficit is probably the most important key in reaching and maintaining the elimination of IDD.

6. Research needs

Elimination of iodine deficiency requires 1) developing simple, qualitative tests to verify inexpensively the level of iodine in salt, rather than indicate only its presence or absence; 2) establishing the best practices of small-scale salt iodization, and simplifying and standardizing the process with appropriate quality assurance; 3) evaluating the impact of using iodized salt in food processing (such as pickling or cheese-making or in various types of cooking) to address the common perceptions of its negative qualities in such processes or inordinately high iodine losses; 4) evaluating factors that have led to successful implementation of IDD programmes so that these can be replicated in areas where progress is lagging or be used to model success in other nutrition or public health programmes.

7. Status of elimination/eradication efforts to date

In 1990, following the World Summit for Children, heads of state and governments of over 120 countries committed themselves to virtually eliminate IDD by the year 2000. UNICEF, other United Nations agencies, and bilateral donors agreed to a mid-decade goal of universal salt iodization. In September 1996, Bolivia was the first country to declare that it had achieved the "virtual elimination of IDD".

Although tremendous progress has been made in most developing countries towards producing iodized salt, substantial gaps remain. The most significant is in the countries of the former Soviet Union, where salt was once partially iodized but by the end of 1997 was largely noniodized. Goitre rates in schoolchildren are high, and cretinism is reported to be serious among newborns in the Central Asian Republics. IDD is serious and not addressed in countries/areas where political control or external access is limited (e.g. China (Autonomous Region of Tibet), Sudan, Afghanistan, and Democratic People's Republic of Korea). Ensuring the correct quantity of iodine in each batch or packet of salt remains a significant problem in many places. The overall adequate quality-assurance programmes are generally lacking in most countries. IDD has re-emerged as a continuing concern in western Europe.

8. Principle challenges to elimination/eradication

Challenges to elimination include 1) raising the level of awareness of the nature and significance of IDD so that governments, salt producers, and others invest in their own protection; 2) ensuring participation by all countries and all regions within countries in the elimination efforts; 3) developing the best manufacturing practices for all salt producers and developing monitoring systems to ensure compliance and eliminate the black market for noniodized salt; 4) developing and maintaining a monitoring system to ensure protection from IDD and employ warning systems to detect breakdowns in salt iodization, or in other protective measures.

Iron deficiency*

1. Brief description of the condition/disease

Iron is critical to the formation of haemoglobin in red blood cells. Iron deficiency and its adverse health consequences result primarily from a dietary iron intake that is inadequate to meet the relatively high iron requirements of young children and reproductive-aged women. In addition, increased blood loss from conditions such as hookworm infection can contribute to iron deficiency.

Anaemia is the most widely recognized consequence of iron deficiency. Severe anaemia can cause death in young children and pregnant women by hindering sufficient oxygen transport to body tissues. In mild-to-moderate anaemia, the most important consequence for adults is reduced work capacity, which can adversely affect the economic output of both families and countries. For young children, the most important consequence of iron deficiency is reduced mental development and cognitive function, potentially aggravated by an increased tendency to absorb lead. For pregnant women, iron-deficiency anaemia is associated with an increased risk of preterm births, which in turn affects child survival and development.

2. Current global burden and ranking within the overall burden of disease

Iron deficiency is a global nutritional problem, affecting primarily infants, children, and reproductive-aged women, especially during pregnancy. Using anaemia as an indicator of iron deficiency, an estimated 50–60% of young children, 20–30% of nonpregnant women, and 50–60% of pregnant women in developing countries are iron deficient. In developed countries, approximately 5% of young children and 5–10% of reproductive-aged women are affected.

In a recent review based on 22 studies from Africa and Asia, anaemia accounted for approximately 20% of maternal mortality. In Africa, 30% of childhood mortality also is associated with severe anaemia. The average reduction in cognitive performance related to iron-deficiency anaemia approximates one standard deviation of the scale used to assess intellectual development. For adults who suffer from iron-deficiency anaemia, the reduction in work productivity is approximately 10–15% depending on the severity of anaemia. For populations where 30% of women and 10% of men have significant anaemia, the net loss of productivity approximates 2–3% of the gross domestic product (GDP).

3. Feasibility (biological) of elimination/eradication

Nutrition education has generally been ineffective in addressing iron deficiency because food from animal sources, which contains more bioavailable iron, is often not affordable by the poor. Iron supplementation for pregnant women is common, but its effectiveness is limited because it requires a functional distribution system and adequate communication to women, which is not feasible in many settings. In many areas where iron-deficiency anaemia is severe, supplementation is not sufficient to meet the high iron requirements of pregnancy. Supplementation for younger children and nonpregnant women can be justified, but the cost and logistics for long-term supplementation make this a difficult proposition.

The most viable approach to control iron-deficiency anaemia is through fortification of major food commodities. This is particularly feasible in areas where cereal products, such as wheat flour, are centrally processed and where the food to be fortified is frequently consumed. Up to 60 mg of iron can be added to each kg of wheat or corn flour, and can provide up to 30% of the daily iron requirement in areas where consumption of the fortified food item is high. In countries where fortification of commonly consumed foods is feasible, iron deficiency can be eliminated or substantially reduced, particularly among people with relatively low iron requirements, such as schoolaged children and nonpregnant women. The recent experience with iron fortification in Venezuela provides an example.

For pregnant women, fortification *per se* is not sufficient, and supplementation is still needed to prevent maternal anaemia. Because their diet often differs from that of adults, infants and young children may benefit little from a general fortification programme, unless their diet is specifically fortified with iron. The effectiveness of targeted fortification was demonstrated in Chile, where fortification of government-distributed milk powder for infants re-

* Contributed by Ray Yip, UNICEF, New York, USA.

sulted in the elimination of iron-deficiency anaemia. Through such measures, a substantial reduction in iron-deficiency anaemia is feasible, but virtual elimination is difficult to achieve among those with high iron requirements, such as pregnant women. In tropical areas where hookworm infection is common and intense, periodic deworming of older children and adults is essential to reduce the burden of severe anaemia related to iron deficiency. Deworming is feasible through school-based programmes and, for pregnant women, through maternal and child health services.

4. Estimated costs and benefits of elimination/eradication

In general, the cost of fortification is very low. For areas with high consumption of wheat flour (e.g. 50 kg per person per year), the cost of added iron is about US$ 0.05 per person per year, and there is no additional cost to deliver the iron to the consumer. For practical purposes the cost of iron fortification of major commodities is low — less than 0.3% of the cost of the wheat flour. Such costs can easily be absorbed by the consumer without input from the public sector. In the case of iron supplements for pregnant women, the cost of a 120-day supply of iron tablets is only about US$ 0.40, but there are substantial costs to the health system for distribution and communication. On a population basis, an overall average cost of US$ 0.20 per person per year would provide for fortification of infant diets, targeted supplementation, fortification of one or more major food commodities, and deworming for older children and reproductive-aged women through schools, work sites, and family planning systems.

A comprehensive programme of this type could reduce iron-deficiency anaemia by up to 80%. The net savings from improved work productivity could be US$ 10 per capita for a country with a per capita GDP of US$ 500, representing 2% of GDP; this gives a cost-effectiveness ratio of 50. However, the benefit of an 80% reduction of iron-deficiency anaemia would include better child development and learning capacity, less morbidity and mortality, and thus reduced direct health-care costs. Even though these human resources are difficult to estimate, it is not unreasonable to assume that taking these additional benefits could double the cost-effectiveness ratio from 50 to 100. The World Bank recently estimated the ratio at 500. Even if the cost-effectiveness ratio is conservatively estimated at 100, the elimination of iron deficiency is still a bargain.

5. Key strategies to accomplish the objective

A comprehensive approach is needed to address iron deficiency as outlined below.

• For infants, a feasible means to improve the quality of complementary feeding needs to be defined. The consumption of foods from animal sources also needs to be increased. This approach can be considered in some settings because the amounts required for infants are relatively small, and hence are potentially affordable. Explore the possible fortification of common food items in the infant diet that are industrially processed, and in the absence of a dietary approach, consider supplementation of infants with iron from 6 to 12 months.

• For schoolchildren and women of reproductive age, consider iron fortification of a common staple food, such as wheat flour or fish sauce. Implement deworming in areas where hookworm is a significant burden. Implement periodic, supervised supplementation in settings where this is feasible, such as schools.

• For pregnant women, improve the supplementation programme by assuring the availability of iron tablets. Provide for adequate education and communication to both health workers and women on the indications for iron supplements to prevent anaemia.

• For all target groups, include other micronutrients. In developing countries, iron deficiency is usually not an isolated nutritional deficit. Low intake of food from animal sources also results in deficiencies in zinc, calcium, riboflavin, and vitamin A. Some of these deficiencies, such as vitamin A deficiency, also contribute to anaemia. For this reason, fortification or supplementation efforts to improve iron status should not be restricted to iron.

6. Research needs

• Develop a low-cost micronutrient additive in the form of sprinkles or drops for complementary foods for infants which can be added to food prepared at home. This strategy could be considered for areas that have no means to improve the infant diet using local or centrally processed fortified foods.

• Develop a low-cost iron complex for supplementation or fortification instead of using the more reactive iron salt. Currently available iron complexes are expensive for large-scale applications, although the amounts required are less and increased market opportunities for such compounds would probably decrease the costs.

• Support the development of cereal grains that have greater bioavailability of iron.

7. Status of elimination/eradication efforts to date

Progress in eliminating iron deficiency has been limited. In 1990 the World Summit for Children called for a one-third reduction in maternal anaemia by the year 2000. However, only in the last 2 years has the importance of preventing iron-deficiency anaemia for young children become an issue, especially through the efforts of UNICEF and USAID. Greatest progress has been made in South and Central America, where several countries have initiated iron fortification of wheat flour. In Asia and Africa, the effort is lagging. Thus far, the USA and Chile are the only countries to have documented the near elimination of childhood iron-deficiency anaemia resulting from widespread use of iron-fortified milk powder or formula. This is likely to be the case for many European countries, but data are lacking to assess whether childhood iron-deficiency anaemia has been eliminated.

8. Principle challenges to elimination/eradication

• To address effectively the problem of maternal anaemia, methods must be found to provide improved baseline iron status to women *before* pregnancy. Because current interventions are overly focused within the health sector, nutrition and health experts need to communicate effectively with the private sector and the food industry because fortification is necessarily an industry-based approach.

• Preventing iron-deficiency anaemia during late infancy and early childhood needs to be addressed. In many settings, this means improving complementary feeding practices. Efforts to address iron deficiency must include control of other micronutrient deficiencies because poor diets cause multiple deficiencies that affect the health of children.

• Policy-makers must be willing to accept solutions or approaches that do not necessarily target all groups or all segments of the population simultaneously, because a single strategy is unlikely to prevent iron deficiency in all populations at risk. Although interventions should be part of a comprehensive strategy, simultaneous implementation of all aspects of the strategy might not be feasible.

Vitamin A deficiency*

1. Brief description of the condition/disease

Vitamin A deficiency is defined by tissue concentrations of vitamin A low enough to have adverse health consequences even if there is no evidence of clinical deficiency (xerophthalmia). Subclinical deficiency is defined by serum retinol levels <0.70 μmol/l, which are considered of moderate and severe public health significance when the prevalence in a population is >10% and >20%, respectively. The consequences of subclinical deficiency are increased risk of mortality from common childhood infections, such as diarrhoea and measles, and recent studies suggest increased risk of maternal mortality. Xerophthalmia occurs when ocular signs are present, including night blindness, Bitot's spots with conjunctival xerosis, and corneal xerosis (which are potentially reversible signs), and keratomalacia, which can result in partial or total irreversible blindness.

2. Current global burden and rating within the overall burden of disease

Approximately 3 million children develop xerophthalmia annually, 250000 to 500000 of whom become blind, and at least 60% die within one year. Estimates of subclinical deficiency among preschool-aged children range from 75 million to 250 million. Recently reported studies from Nepal suggest that in South Asia alone, 1–2 million pregnant women may be at risk from subclinical vitamin A deficiency.

3. Feasibility (biological) of elimination/eradication

Eliminating vitamin A deficiency and all its consequences, including blindness, as a public health problem is feasible if dietary intake is increased to the recommended levels through natural foods, fortified foods, and/or supplements, and if the burden of other infectious diseases, which exacerbate vitamin A deficiency and lower serum retinol levels, is re-

* Contributed by Barbara A. Underwood, Food and Nutrition Board, Institute of Medicine, National Academy of Sciences, Washington, DC 20418, USA.

duced. It is unlikely that vitamin A deficiency will be eradicated because it is caused by an inadequate dietary intake for economic, social, or cultural reasons, some of which are based on individual human behaviour and choice. However, elimination can be monitored by the prevalence of low serum levels.

4. Estimated costs and benefits of elimination/eradication

The cost of elimination depends on the mix of intervention strategies selected for implementation. After the initial capital investment costs, fortification of a staple food is a long-term low-cost intervention. Vitamin A supplements are inexpensive — less than US$ 0.03 per capsule — but costs for delivery may be high depending on the infrastructures used. Semi-annual campaigns have proven cost-effective and achieved broad coverage. Similarly, linking the distribution of capsules to vaccination delivery systems has reduced delivery costs. Dietary modification to increase the quantity and quality of menus depends on physical and economic access to food sources and educational/social marketing to guide food choice behaviours. Expected societal benefits include reduced costs for use of medical resources by reduced disease severity and individual benefits of reduced risk of death.

5. Key strategies to accomplish the objectives

A combination of strategies addressing short- and long-term needs is usually required for sustainable control and elimination. These strategies include direct measures to increase intake of vitamin A through food, such as dietary modification in terms of quantity and quality, fortification, and supplementation; and indirect measures through public health strategies to control disease; income-generating activities to increase buying power; and the empowerment of women through the use of strategies such as literacy and education programmes. The emphasis given to each of the strategies depends on the severity of the problem. Also, increased political and public awareness of the problem, its consequences, and potential solutions is essential to obtain the needed commitment to elimination from national to community levels. Because preschool-aged children and pregnant and lactating women are those who are the most vulnerable to deficiency consequences, strategies should focus first on meeting their short-term needs, perhaps through supplementation, while the longer-term control measures — dietary modification and fortification — are concurrently being established.

6. Research needs

Research is needed to develop a reliable, low-cost, field-applicable indicator or methodologies for diagnosing subclinical deficiency and monitoring control strategies (this is a priority because serum retinol values are expensive, subject to confounding, and not a reliable index of vitamin A status of individuals except at extremes); assess the bioavailability of carotenoids from typical menus eaten by children in areas with endemic deficiency; conduct operational research to determine the safety and feasibility of community-controlled frequent distribution of low-dose supplements to young children and pregnant women; and develop simple, community-based technology for fortification programmes, either with vitamin A fortificants or through food-to-food combinations using concentrated food sources added to common low-vitamin-A diets of children and pregnant women (e.g. dried mangoes, dark green leafy vegetables or yellow squash added to complementary and post-weaning paps and cereals).

7. Status of elimination/eradication efforts to date

In the past decade, great strides have been made in identifying populations at risk of deficiency, reducing the prevalence of xerophthalmia, and planning and implementing intervention strategies. Baseline information is available for most countries with a problem. It is too soon after implementation to evaluate fully the impact of various intervention strategies on a global basis. Where this has been possible on a national or subnational basis, horticulture, fortification, and supplementation strategies are all effective when coverage of the vulnerable population is high. Public health measures and other indirect measures contribute to making direct intake strategies more effective and efficient. In addition, more political awareness exists of the problem and commitment to its elimination is more widespread than in any previous period.

8. Principal challenges to elimination/eradication

The principal challenges include the following:

— sustaining global and national commitment to elimination;

— embedding successful control strategies into community systems so that they are sustained;

— increasing dietary intakes of young children and fertile women to adequate levels; and

— educating the medical profession and general public, especially mothers, about the need for vitamin A and its locally available sources for menu planning.

2. Bacterial diseases

Congenital syphilis*

1. Brief description of the condition/disease

Congenital syphilis results from infection of the fetus by *Treponema pallidum*, the causative agent of syphilis. During the first 4 years after acquiring syphilis, an untreated pregnant woman has a >70% probability of transmitting the infection to her fetus. About 40% of pregnancies in women with untreated early syphilis end in perinatal death. Infected live born infants can develop acute systemic illness, bone deformities, developmental disabilities, blindness, or deafness. Only about 50% of infected neonates will immediately manifest these serious problems, with others developing them later in life. Congenital syphilis can be prevented if infected pregnant women are treated with penicillin. However, the painless genital sores of primary syphilis frequently go unnoticed by women, and they do not seek care. In areas where coverage of prenatal care is low, women do not receive routine syphilis testing during pregnancy. Furthermore, increasingly strong evidence indicates that syphilis, like other causes of genital ulcers, greatly enhances HIV transmission, making prevention of syphilis in women additionally important for control of HIV infection. The occurrence of congenital syphilis represents a failure in the basic systems of sexually transmitted disease (STD) control and prenatal care.

2. Current global burden and rating within the overall burden of disease

Congenital syphilis remains one of the most severe, preventable adverse pregnancy outcomes throughout the world. The World Bank ranks syphilis fifth globally in disability-adjusted life days (DALDs) lost per capita per year, after measles, HIV infection, malaria, and gastroenteritis. Syphilis results in an estimated loss of 16 DALDs per capita per year in the developing world, and to the extent that syphilis enhances HIV transmission, an additional 61 DALDs per capita per year. Estimated syphilis-associated disability-adjusted life years (DALYs) lost among children aged <5 years are 500 000 per year; additional DALYs are lost for older children and adults from persistent physical and developmental disabilities.

In 1995, WHO estimated that the worldwide annual incidence of sexually acquired syphilis was 0.4% (12 million cases) and that prevalence was 1% (28 million cases). Given the estimated 6 million incident syphilis infections among women annually, that 90% of these are among women of reproductive age, and that the fertility rate is 20% per year, approximately 900 000 gestations occur annually among infected women. An estimated 40% of these pregnancies (360 000) end in fetal or perinatal death, and 50% of the remaining neonates (270 000) suffer significant physical, developmental, and sensory impairments.

3. Feasibility (biological) of elimination

Syphilis elimination is biologically feasible because no naturally occurring nonhuman host exists for the disease, serological tests for diagnosis are relatively accurate (>95% sensitive and specific), and curative treatment is available — early syphilis can be treated with a single injection of penicillin. The biological feasibility of syphilis elimination (including the elimination of congenital syphilis) has been demonstrated in most of the developed world. For example, in the USA, the widespread availability of penicillin in the mid-1940s and the targeted control efforts of the U.S. Public Health Service resulted in a 93% decline in primary and secondary syphilis over 10 years, from a rate of 60 per 100 000 population in 1945 to only 4 per 100 000 population in 1955. Congenital syphilis has also declined dramatically in the USA, United Kingdom, and other developed countries during the past 50 years, as a result of prenatal syphilis screening and treatment.

* Contributed by Lyn Finelli, Stuart M. Berman, Emilia H. Koumans, and William C. Levine, Centers for Disease Control and Prevention, Atlanta, GA, USA.

4. Estimated costs and benefits of elimination

The country-specific costs of effective congenital syphilis elimination campaigns depend on the prevalence of syphilis in the population, the coverage and quality of prenatal care, and basic public health measures for STD control. In countries with a 1% syphilis prevalence, the estimated costs of antenatal screening and treatment programmes are US$ 0.42 per pregnant woman, and of averting each syphilis-associated adverse pregnancy outcome, US$ 70; in countries with a 15% prevalence, estimated costs are US$ 0.70 and US$ 9.28, respectively. PAHO estimates that an elimination programme in the Region of the Americas would cost US$ 400 000 each year to coordinate, with an additional $100 000 needed in each Member State. The cost of an elimination programme may be substantially higher in sub-Saharan Africa, where the prevalence of syphilis is higher and the coverage of prenatal and STD services is less.

Congenital syphilis contributes to as many as 29% of perinatal and infant deaths, 26% of stillbirths, 11% of neonatal deaths, and 5% of postneonatal deaths. In addition to preventing this morbidity, an elimination programme that implements the strategies described below would confer far-reaching collateral benefits by supporting improvements in prenatal care and HIV-prevention programmes. Even without considering the impact on HIV transmission, cure or prevention of a single case of syphilis saves 161 DALYs; when the contribution of syphilis to HIV transmission is also considered, 396 DALYs per cured or prevented case are saved.

5. Key strategies to accomplish the objective

Strategies for eliminating congenital syphilis (adapted from PAHO) include the following:

— strengthening surveillance;

— improving procedures for syphilis testing of pregnant women by using simple and rapid serological tests that are already available; and

— enhancing the capacity of prenatal care services to identify and manage cases of maternal syphilis.

These should be complemented by strategies that would improve the control of syphilis (and other STDs) in high-risk populations and by syndromic management of genital ulcers, as advocated by WHO and UNAIDS. In countries with high rates of syphilis, congenital syphilis elimination will require that syphilis rates are reduced (but not necessarily eliminated) in high-prevalence populations. A programme of congenital syphilis elimination that includes targeted efforts for high prevalence populations will also prevent HIV infection. Strategies that result in strong partnerships with both the reproductive health and the HIV prevention communities have the best chances for success.

6. Research needs

In each country, operations research will be needed to develop new paradigms for the transition from syphilis control to elimination, to determine the optimal balance among the different strategies described, and to identify approaches to implement these strategies and to overcome obstacles. For example, in some countries it may be necessary to identify physical, social and cultural barriers to prenatal care. When barriers are identified, further studies may be needed to evaluate practical interventions. The cost-effectiveness of congenital syphilis prevention in traditional and non-traditional health care settings (i.e. in prenatal clinics versus rural areas with lay caregivers) should also be evaluated. Finally, research is needed to evaluate potential one-dose oral treatments and rapid, non-invasive syphilis tests; fingerstick testing methods and one-step strip testing using *T. pallidum*-specific recombinant antigens are available, but further field testing is needed to develop quality control methods and assess their usefulness.

7. Status of elimination efforts to date

In 1995, all PAHO Member States resolved to eliminate congenital syphilis in the Americas. Their goal is to reduce congenital syphilis to ≤0.5 cases per 1000 births by detecting and treating over 95% of infected pregnant women and reducing the overall prevalence of syphilis during pregnancy to <1%. Since this resolution, systematic efforts towards elimination, including the development of comprehensive plans have taken place in several Member States, including Argentina, Bolivia, Brazil, and Colombia. Mothercare, a USAID-funded organization, has developed a training package for syphilis prevention and control in maternal and child-health programmes, which has been field-tested in Latin America and Africa and provided to more than 30 countries. Recently, progress in programme development has been reported from Nairobi, Kenya, where syphilis screening of pregnant women increased from 60% to 100% and treatment from 9% to 85%. A programme in Lusaka, Zambia, documented a 50% reduction in adverse pregnancy outcomes over several years by increasing maternal syphilis screening and maternal and partner treatment.

8. Principal challenges to congenital syphilis elimination

Despite the impact of congenital syphilis on maternal and infant health, and the demonstrated biologi-
cal feasibility of elimination, it was not until PAHO developed its elimination programme in 1995 that this condition began to receive increasing recognition by governments and donor agencies. Among the principal challenges to the elimination of congenital syphilis are the lack of awareness and understanding of the problem by persons involved in maternal and child health programmes and in HIV prevention programmes. Building support among the many organizations and public health professionals working in these areas will be critical if we are to mount a global effort to eliminate this disease.

Diphtheria*

1. Brief description of the condition/disease

Before the development of a vaccine, diphtheria was a major cause of morbidity and mortality among children in temperate climates, especially in crowded urban areas, even after the introduction of an antitoxin in the 1890s reduced the mortality for severe cases from 25–50% to 5–10%.

Diphtheria is caused by toxigenic strains of *Corynebacterium diphtheriae*; these strains carry a phage coding for the toxin and are transmitted from human to human primarily by infected secretions from the respiratory tract and skin lesions. Absorption of the toxin causes severe tissue damage locally in the respiratory tract, heart, and peripheral nerves, resulting in fatalities due to obstruction of the airway, myocarditis, and diffuse polyneuritis.

2. Current global burden and rating within the overall burden of disease

Almost complete elimination of diphtheria has been noted in developed countries after childhood vaccination coverage against diphtheria reached 70–80%. Many European countries have not reported cases in more than a decade; almost all the rare cases in others are linked to known importation. In the USA during 1980–95, only 41 cases were reported, and all except one of the culture-proven cases since 1990 were linked to known importation. Low incidence and lack of epidemics persist in these countries despite the gradual accumulation of large numbers of adults who are susceptible because of waning vaccine-induced immunity.

Many developing countries do not have reliable incidence data on diphtheria because of the need for laboratory diagnosis and good surveillance systems. However, the disease burden appears much smaller for diphtheria than for measles or diarrhoeal disease. Cases reported from developing countries have decreased dramatically as coverage with three doses of DPT (DPT3) increased (from 46% in 1985 to 79% in 1992), accounting for most of the global decrease during the 1970s and 1980s (77 040 cases in 1974 and 23 557 in 1988).

However, during the 1990s, diphtheria has resurged in both developed and developing countries where it had been well controlled. An epidemic that began in 1990 in the Newly Independent States (NIS) of the former USSR caused almost 150 000 reported cases and 5000 deaths by the end of 1996. Before aggressive vaccination campaigns during the epidemic, coverage of DPT3 was <80% among infants and <25% for receipt of a booster dose among adults. Overall, most reported cases and fatalities occurred in adults. Control has been achieved in most NIS by achieving unprecedented levels of adult immunization in addition to intensifying childhood immunization. Developing countries, such as Ecuador (approximately 400 cases in 1993–94) and Algeria (approximately 1000 cases in 1992–96), have also reported outbreaks after periods of good control following implementation of childhood immunization programmes.

Circulation of toxigenic strains of *C. diphtheriae* persists in parts of both developed and developing countries where diphtheria is not being reported. For example, a focus of toxigenic *C. diphtheriae* was found in South Dakota in 1996 with molecular analysis of strains suggesting local persistence since the 1970s; and a recent serological study in rural Kenya showed high diphtheria immunity among unvaccinated persons, suggesting continued circulation.

3. Feasibility (biological) of elimination/eradication

Eradication is not currently feasible because preliminary evidence suggests that circulation of toxigenic *C. diphtheriae* might persist, even in populations with fairly high childhood immunization coverage, and might be difficult to detect; and sustainable reservoirs for the toxin gene might exist in nonhuman mammals. Future feasibility depends on understanding prevention of continued circulation and evidence that circulation of the toxin gene in the animal reservoirs is not sustained indefinitely.

Four factors favour eradication: humans are the only known sustained reservoir; an inexpensive and safe toxoid vaccine exists; high coverage with this vaccine appears to reduce circulation of toxigenic strains of *C. diphtheriae* in the human population and to prevent disease; and seasonality exists for both respiratory and cutaneous diphtheria, making transmission of toxigenic strains more vulnerable to interruption.

* Contributed by Charles Vitek and Jay Wenger, Centers for Disease Control and Prevention, Atlanta, GA, USA.

Seven factors could hinder eradication: the phage carrying the toxin gene can occasionally be found in nondiphtheria *Corynebacterium* species infecting animals (this may represent an ineradicable reservoir for reintroduction of toxin gene into non-toxigenic *C. diphtheriae* strains); infection with a toxigenic strain can either be direct or *in situ* by a phage carrying the toxin gene, infecting a commensal non-toxigenic *C. diphtheriae* strain; an asymptomatic carrier state exists, even among immune persons, and circulation appears to be able to continue under some settings, even in populations with fairly high childhood immunization rates; immunity to diphtheria is not life-long (a minimum of three doses is required for effective primary immunization, and periodic booster doses are required throughout adult life to maintain protective titres — in addition, immune persons are not distinguishable from susceptible persons except by serological or Schick testing; in countries with low incidence, both the clinician and the laboratory can easily miss the diagnosis of diphtheria, and empirical antibiotic treatment can prevent recovery of the organism; limited epidemiological, clinical, and laboratory expertise is available on diphtheria; and political will may be lacking because the disease burden is low in developed countries and is perceived to be relatively low in developing countries.

4. Estimated costs and benefits of elimination/eradication

Near elimination could be achieved with full implementation of EPI. Benefits of diphtheria elimination are difficult to estimate in the absence of good data on disease burden in many developing countries. Developed countries would have fewer imported cases. The benefits of full implementation of EPI would extend to the other childhood diseases. Because an effective strategy for eradication is unknown, costs have not yet been calculated.

5. Key strategies to accomplish the objectives

For elimination, implementation of the EPI programme (>90% coverage with DPT3), coupled with childhood boosters, might allow near elimination of the disease. Maintenance of the disease-free state could require some level of coverage of the adult population (as suggested by the recent epidemic in the NIS).

For eradication, high coverage and high socioeconomic standards in many temperate-zone countries appear to have interrupted circulation of toxigenic *C. diphtheriae*. It is unclear whether this strategy is applicable to developing countries, especially those with lower socioeconomic conditions.

6. Research needs

For elimination, knowledge is needed of the level of vaccine-induced immunity among both children and adults which is sufficient to prevent circulation of toxigenic strains in the population and to provide herd immunity in both developed and developing countries. In addition, knowledge is needed of the epidemiological effect of widespread vaccination in developing countries.

For eradication, knowledge is needed about whether carriage of the toxin gene among zoonotic *Corynebacterium* strains is stable enough to make eradication impossible and the factors that allow persistent circulation of toxigenic strains despite fairly high levels of childhood vaccination.

7. Status of elimination/eradication efforts to date

Implementation of EPI has achieved remarkable progress in decreasing the burden of disease in countries where reliable data are collected.

8. Principal challenges to elimination/eradication

The principal challenges to elimination are lack of adequate data about the schedule of childhood and adult boosters which can prevent the disease reliably, and difficulties in global implementation of EPI and the necessary booster schedules.

The principal challenges to eradication are lack of data that toxigenic *C. diphtheriae* can be eradicated with the current vaccine under the present socioeconomic conditions in which much of the global population lives, and lack of consensus that diphtheria is an important problem globally.

Haemophilus influenzae type B infection*

1. Brief description of the condition/disease

Haemophilus influenzae type b (Hib) is a bacterium that causes meningitis, pneumonia, septicaemia, and other severe, invasive infections. Meningitis is characterized by infection of the spinal fluid and the meninges, a membrane that surrounds the brain. In the USA and other developed countries, approximately 5% of patients with meningitis die, and up to 30% of survivors have long-term disabilities ranging from hearing loss to severe mental retardation. In developing countries, up to 50% of Hib patients die in some settings.

2. Current global burden and rating within the overall burden of disease

In the absence of vaccination, Hib was consistently identified as the leading cause of bacterial meningitis among under-5-year-olds in developed countries. Before vaccination in the USA, an estimated 1 of every 200 children had an invasive Hib infection before the age 5 years. In developing countries, Hib is the leading cause of bacterial meningitis-associated deaths and the second leading cause of bacterial pneumonia deaths. Globally, Hib meningitis and pneumonia cause 380 000–500 000 deaths among under-5-year-olds each year. Accurate Hib disease incidence data are lacking for many parts of Asia and the Pacific Rim.

3. Feasibility (biological) of elimination/eradication

The biological feasibility of Hib eradication is difficult to determine, but several aspects of Hib disease and Hib vaccines make elimination possible. Hib is a uniquely human pathogen with no known reservoir in the environment. Hib polysaccharide-protein conjugate vaccines are highly effective (efficacy of 90–100%) in preventing disease, and should provide long-lasting protection. Hib conjugate vaccines also can interrupt transmission by preventing asymptomatic carriage and are thereby able to protect unvaccinated persons through herd immunity. At the practical level, Hib conjugate vaccines are still too expensive for many countries to use, they require more than one dose to provide substantial protection, and not all countries may be able to achieve the levels of vaccination coverage needed for elimination. Thus, programmatic obstacles are the major barriers to elimination.

The feasibility of eradicating Hib is more difficult to determine. At the molecular level, eliminating the genetic material that codes for the type b capsule is more difficult than eliminating the apparent occurrence of type b infections. With more research into the molecular biology of Hib and further experience with the vaccines, it may be possible to determine more accurately the feasibility of eradication.

4. Estimated costs and benefits of elimination/eradication

Although economic analyses of programmes to eliminate/eradicate Hib have not been carried out, a recent analysis of the cost-effectiveness of routine Hib vaccination globally determined that, at current vaccination coverage rates, such a programme could prevent 58–83% of all Hib-related deaths and Hib-related disability-adjusted life years (DALY) lost at a cost of US$ 35–53 per DALY saved. This cost-per-DALY saved compares favourably with other new immunizations and with other life-saving interventions. The analysis, however, assumed that vaccine could be purchased at US$ 1 per dose, a price that should be attainable but is still lower than the current price.

5. Key strategies to accomplish the objective(s)

Routine vaccination through national programmes is the cornerstone of control of Hib disease. Efforts to maintain high coverage and timely vaccination will improve the effectiveness of this control strategy. Ensuring a steady, affordable supply of Hib vaccine for developing countries will be essential. Efforts

* Contributed by Orin Levine, Jay Wenger, Yand Bradley Perkins, Nancy Rosenstein and Anne Schuchat, Centers for Disease Control and Prevention, Atlanta, GA, USA, and the Global Programme for Vaccines, WHO, Geneva, Switzerland.

to eliminate Hib in countries with moderate-to-poor vaccination coverage will depend on the ability of the Hib vaccination programme to interrupt transmission and thereby provide herd immunity. Whether routine Hib vaccination will result in herd immunity in developing countries is still unclear. Further experience with Hib vaccines in developing countries may provide insights to novel strategies for maximizing the herd immunity effects of vaccination. Surveillance for Hib disease, including laboratory identification of the bacterium, will be required to monitor the impact of vaccination.

6. Research needs

Because experience with Hib conjugate vaccines is relatively limited (about 10 years), continued assessment is needed of the long-term impact on immunity and on carriage rates. The mechanism for interrupting Hib transmission is still unknown. Continued efforts on new and improved Hib vaccines, which may be less expensive or provide immunity with fewer doses, are warranted. Additionally, research is needed to determine if it is possible to eradicate the gene for the type b capsule from populations of *H. influenzae* bacteria.

Because an accurate surveillance programme with relatively simple diagnostic methods would be critical during an eradication campaign, a non-invasive test for confirmation of Hib meningitis should be developed. Such a sentinel test should be supplemented with a standardized protocol to quantify the associated impact on Hib carriage.

In many countries, particularly in Asia, the burden of Hib disease remains largely undefined. Because the political will to pursue vaccination will depend in large part on the magnitude of the Hib disease burden locally, additional efforts are needed to quantify the burden of Hib disease where it remains undefined.

7. Status of elimination/eradication efforts to date

The widespread use of Hib conjugate vaccines for routine vaccination of infants and young children has dramatically reduced the incidence of the disease and the transmission of Hib organisms in several developed countries. In the Nordic countries (Finland, Iceland, Sweden, Norway, and Denmark) routine vaccination has essentially eliminated Hib disease, and in Finland and Iceland carriage in young children is no longer detected. In the USA, the impact of Hib vaccination has been equally dramatic: the incidence of Hib disease in young children has declined by >95%, and good evidence exists that Hib vaccination has interrupted transmission and protected unvaccinated children by herd immunity. In developing countries, however, where the epidemiology of Hib disease differs substantially from the epidemiology in the USA and Europe, the impact of widespread vaccination is still unclear.

8. Principal challenges to elimination/eradication

The current price of Hib conjugate vaccines is the principal obstacle to the wider control of Hib disease globally. Efforts to ensure access to a steady, inexpensive supply of vaccine will be needed. Hib vaccines combined with other newer vaccines having a broader impact on meningitis and acute respiratory infections may be more acceptable. A lack of information on the burden of disease in some regions also limits the vaccine's uptake in some regions that can afford it. Elimination of Hib invasive disease may be possible in the future, but additional experience with the use of Hib conjugate vaccines for control of Hib disease in nonindustrialized countries will be needed before the feasibility of eradication can be evaluated adequately.

Leprosy*

1. Brief description of the disease

Leprosy is a chronic infectious disease caused by *Mycobacterium leprae*. It usually affects the skin and peripheral nerves but has a wide range of possible clinical manifestations. The disease is classified as paucibacillary or multibacillary leprosy (i.e. tuberculoid or lepromatous leprosy, respectively). Paucibacillary leprosy is a milder disease characterized by one or more hypopigmented, hypoaesthic skin lesions. Multibacillary leprosy is associated with symmetric skin lesions, nodules, plaques, thickened dermis, and frequent involvement of the nasal mucosa resulting in nasal congestion and epistaxis, and of peripheral nerve trunks resulting in deformities of the limbs, eyes and face.

The mode of transmission of leprosy remains uncertain but most investigators believe *M. leprae* is usually spread from person to person primarily as a nasal droplet infection. The incubation period is unusually long for a bacterial disease, generally 5–7 years, with the shortest period being 2–3 years and the longest up to 40 years. Peak age of onset is young adulthood, usually 20–30 years of age; disease is rarely seen in children under 5 years of age.

Leprosy is usually diagnosed by its clinical manifestations, which are characterized by anaesthetic skin lesions and inflammation of peripheral nerve trunks. The diagnosis is confirmed by skin biopsy and acid-fast staining, which are also used to stage disease and judge the response to therapy. Since 1982, WHO has advocated use of multidrug therapy (MDT) regimens to treat paucibacillary leprosy (6 months) and multibacillary leprosy (12 months). This regimen has served as the cornerstone for elimination efforts.

2. Current global burden and rating within the overall burden of disease

In 1985, WHO estimated 10–12 million leprosy cases worldwide; 5.4 million of these were registered in a leprosy programme. At the beginning of 1998, WHO reported that 883 340 were registered and being treated. Another 1–2 million people are permanently disabled as a result of leprosy but are considered free of active infection.

Each year, an estimated 500 000 new leprosy cases are identified. Most come from 32 countries where the disease continues to be considered a public health problem. At the beginning of 1998, 16 countries — Bangladesh, Brazil, Cambodia, Democratic Republic of the Congo, Ethiopia, Guinea, India, Indonesia, Madagascar, Mozambique, Myanmar, Nepal, Niger, Nigeria, Philippines, and Sudan — reported more the 90% of the world's leprosy cases.

3. Feasibility (biological) of elimination/eradication

Elimination of leprosy may be feasible. Although other animals (e.g. armadillos) carry *M. leprae*, humans are believed to be the organism's major reservoir, and MDT is curative. However, prolonged incubation of leprosy makes recognition of a disease-free area difficult. Asymptomatic carriers of *M. leprae* may infect other people, and the frequently chronic and mild symptoms may be difficult to detect without systematic screening of populations.

4. Estimated costs and benefits of elimination/eradication

The estimated cost to identify and treat 2 million leprosy cases per year for the 3 years 1997–2000 is US$ 250 million; drugs account for 10% of the total cost. Prevention of leprosy-associated pain, suffering, ostracism, and disabilities (primarily deformity and blindness) is the primary benefit. In addition, resources now devoted to leprosy treatment and rehabilitation programmes could be directed elsewhere.

5. Key strategies to accomplish the objective

The strategy has focused primarily on increasing case-finding and expanding MDT services to all health facilities; ensuring that all existing and new cases are treated appropriately with MDT; encouraging all patients to take treatment regularly and completely; promoting leprosy awareness in the community so that people with suspicious lesions will report voluntarily for diagnosis and treatment; setting targets and time tables for activities and making all efforts to achieve them; and improving

* Contributed by Richard A. Spiegel and Bradley A. Perkins, Centers for Disease Control and Prevention, Atlanta, GA, USA.

surveillance and tracking of patients to monitor progress towards elimination.

BCG vaccine is effective in preventing leprosy in some populations but its role in leprosy elimination programmes has yet to be defined.

6. Research needs

• Resistance of *M. leprae* to rifampicin, when used alone as monotherapy, has been identified. Since rifampicin is a key drug in the MDT programme, this should be carefully monitored.

• New drug regimens requiring shorter treatment times are needed. Trials of ofloxacin, minocycline, and rifampicin in various dosages and time intervals are ongoing.

• Validation of supervised intermittent therapy options are needed. These may be useful when patients are living in remote settings.

• Better means are needed to identify *M. leprae* infection at the subclinical and early clinical stages, either through direct detection of the organism or indirectly by serological response.

• In the post-elimination phase, surveillance for leprosy will need to be maintained because of its long incubation time.

7. Status of elimination/eradication efforts to date

WHO's year 2000 goal for eliminating leprosy is defined as a reduction in the number of cases to <1 case per 10 000 population. Since 1985, the estimated number of leprosy cases has declined from 10–12 million to under 1 million registered cases in 1998. During the past 10 years, more than 10 million patients have been cured using MDT.

8. Principal challenges to elimination/eradication

The primary challenges to leprosy elimination are: reaching populations that have not yet received MDT services; improving detection of the disease; and providing patients with quality services and drugs free of charge to patients.

Neonatal tetanus*

1. Brief description of the condition/disease

Neonatal tetanus (NT) results from *Clostridium tetani* infection of the umbilical stump at or following delivery of a child born to a mother without sufficient circulating antibodies to protect the infant passively by transplacental transfer. Contamination of the umbilical stump at or following delivery is especially likely in an unattended delivery or a delivery attended by an untrained midwife. In some areas of the world, the cord is cut with an unclean object or the umbilical stump is traditionally covered with contaminated material. In addition, traditional surgeries (e.g. circumcision, uvulectomy) are associated with increased risk, as are mothers with a history of a previously delivered infant with NT.

The average incubation period is 6 days (range: 3–28 days). NT is characterized by generalized stiffness with spasms or convulsions. The case-fatality ratio is ≥80%.

2. Current global burden and rating within the overall burden of disease

NT is a leading cause of childhood mortality in developing countries and is second only to measles among the vaccine-preventable diseases as a cause of childhood mortality. In some developing countries, NT accounts for one fourth of infant mortality and half of neonatal mortality in unimmunized populations. In 1997, an estimated 277 376 neonatal deaths were attributed to NT, with an estimated global mortality rate of 2.1 per 1000 live births.

3. Feasibility (biological) of elimination/eradication

Because tetanus spores are ubiquitous in the environment, eradication is not biologically feasible. "Elimination" (achieving rates <1 per 1000 live births) is feasible only if high levels of coverage with appropriate strategies are achieved (see below).

4. Estimated costs and benefits of elimination

Tetanus prevention through vaccination is highly cost-effective. The median estimated cost-effectiveness of tetanus toxoid (TT) vaccination programmes is US$ 89 (range, US$ 27–205) per case prevented for routine strategies, and US$ 0.21 (range, US$ 0.55–1.71) for the cost per dose of TT administered during mass campaign strategies. These costs do not include the need for certification as part of an elimination strategy.

5. Key strategies to accomplish the objective

The following are key strategies: achieving and maintaining high vaccination coverage levels for at least two doses of potent TT among reproductive-aged women in high-risk areas; promoting clean delivery, cord-care practices, and other surgical procedures performed on neonates (including the following practices shown to reduce risk: handwashing by the delivery attendant, delivery on a clean surface, use of a sterile or clean cutting tool, and application of a topical antimicrobial to the umbilical stump wound); and targeting women with a history of NT in previous infants.

6. Research and evaluation needs

Studies are needed to determine the following: optimum vaccination schedules for high, long-lasting immunity levels; optimum topical antimicrobial practices; operational approaches to monitor the field effectiveness of TT using data on population coverage and maternal vaccination levels among NT cases; safety of iodine as a topical antimicrobial in newborns and type of iodine to be used; safety and effectiveness of sustained-release TT; duration of protection among girls vaccinated during childhood through EPI; and mechanisms for sensitive surveillance.

7. Status of elimination efforts to date

An elimination goal (defined as <1 case per 1000 live births for all districts) has been established.

* Contributed by D. Rebecca Prevots, Centers for Disease Control and Prevention, Atlanta, GA, USA.

During 1980–95, the number of developing countries that have eliminated NT increased from 38 to 97.

8. Principal challenges to elimination

Challenges to elimination include the following: insufficient resources; coordination of efforts by EPI/MCH to achieve all strategies proposed in Section 5 above; achievement of high coverage levels with two or more doses of potent TT among pregnant women; achievement of high coverage levels with two or more doses of potent TT among women of childbearing age; ensuring that doses of TT meet production and quality requirements; development and delivery of culturally appropriate programmes for promoting vaccination of girls and women and clean-cord and post-surgical care in neonates; development of operational approaches to reach and vaccinate, on a priority basis, women with a history of a previous child with NT; lack of effective surveillance and insufficient political will.

Addendum

In June 1998 the Scientific Advisory Group of Experts (SAGE) for WHO recommended that TT be replaced with tetanus–diphthesia Td vaccine.

Pertussis*

1. Brief description of the condition/disease

Pertussis, a highly infectious, vaccine-preventable disease lasting many weeks, is caused by infection with *Bordetella pertussis*, a bacillus first isolated in 1906 by Bordet and Gengou. Pertussis typically manifests as paroxysmal spasms of severe coughing, whooping, and post-tussive vomiting in children. The major complications, including hypoxia, pneumonia, seizures, encephalopathy and malnutrition, are most common among infants and young children. Pertussis is transmitted by direct contact with discharges from respiratory mucous membranes of infected persons and by airborne droplets. Like measles, it is highly contagious, with up to 90% of susceptible household contacts developing clinical disease following exposure to an index case.

2. Current global burden and rating within the overall burden of disease

Pertussis results in high morbidity and mortality in many countries every year. Worldwide, 206 541 cases were reported in 1994, and 80 606 cases were reported in 1995. However, pertussis cases are substantially underreported in most countries. When this was taken into account, approximately 39 million cases of pertussis and 355 000 pertussis-related deaths occurred in 1995. The estimated number of pertussis cases globally was similar to that of measles cases. The estimated number of pertussis-related deaths is one-third of the estimated number of measles-related deaths and 100 000 fewer than deaths caused by neonatal tetanus.

3. Feasibility (biological) of elimination/eradication

Pertussis elimination/eradication does not seem feasible for several reasons: whole-cell and acellular pertussis vaccines are most effective in preventing severe disease and may have little impact on acquisition of infection, preventing mild disease, and decreasing transmission to other individuals; pertussis

vaccines require multiple doses for protection, hence they require a highly organized vaccine delivery system; immunity following vaccination wanes, and in the absence of booster vaccinations in older children and adults, susceptible adolescents and adults will exist; the true burden of disease is not known because underreporting is a major problem in many countries; and pertussis is difficult to diagnose particularly during the catarrhal stage when it is most contagious (therefore, even aggressive outbreak-control strategies are unlikely to contain it).

Adequate herd immunity to block pertussis transmission in a sustained fashion ($>90\%$ level of population immunity may be needed) may not be attainable even with 100% coverage; the efficacy of currently available acellular and whole-cell vaccines is, at best, 90%.

Side-effects associated with whole-cell pertussis vaccines are a major concern among health care providers and parents. Although new acellular pertussis vaccines cause fewer adverse reactions, they are significantly more expensive, especially when resources are limited in many countries.

Because the pathogenesis of *B. pertussis* and factors related to protection against infection are not well known, development of pertussis vaccines that are effective against infection and laboratory diagnosis of pertussis are challenging.

The following factors favour elimination/eradication: humans are the only reservoir for *B. pertussis*; whole-cell and acellular pertussis vaccines are highly effective in preventing severe disease (the introduction and widespread use of whole-cell pertussis vaccines, together with improving socioeconomic conditions, has resulted in a marked decline in reported pertussis incidence in many countries); seasonality exists for pertussis epidemics, making transmission more vulnerable to interruption; and long-term carriage is thought not to occur.

4. Estimated costs and benefits of elimination/eradication

The estimated costs to eliminate or eradicate pertussis are unknown because an effective strategy has not yet been planned. Benefits of elimination or eradication are difficult to estimate in the absence of accurate data on the true disease burden in all age groups in many countries. However, eradication would allow cessation of vaccination against pertussis.

---

* Contributed by Dalya Guris, Peter Strebel and Melinda Wharton, Centers for Disease Control and Prevention, Atlanta, GA, USA.

5. Key strategies to accomplish the objectives

Pertussis can be reduced among children with implementation of the EPI programme (>90% coverage with DPT3) and improved surveillance. However, elimination or eradication strategies have not been established because of limitations listed above in Section 3.

6. Research needs

Research is needed to assess the true burden of infection in all age groups; develop and evaluate vaccines that are efficacious and safe for use among adolescents and adults; develop better diagnostic methods that are more sensitive and easy to perform and yield timely results; demonstrate local or regional elimination and the effectiveness of outbreak-control measures; further laboratory research to understand the pathogenesis of *B. pertussis* and host factors that are associated with protection against infection; and determine transmission patterns and identify critical factors involved in transmission to other persons through epidemiological studies.

7. Status of elimination/eradication efforts to date

Implementation of EPI has achieved remarkable progress in decreasing pertussis incidence in many countries. However, the true burden of disease is difficult to estimate because of problems with diagnosis and reporting of pertussis.

8. Principal challenges to elimination/eradication

Challenges to eliminating/eradicating pertussis are as follows: current vaccines may not prevent infection and transmission to others, and immunity is not lifelong; effective booster vaccination for adolescents and adults is not available; highly sensitive and specific diagnostic tests that are also easy and quick to perform are not available; knowledge of the true disease burden in all age groups is lacking; and implementation of EPI is difficult.

Trachoma*

1. Brief description of the condition/disease

Trachoma is a bacterial disease of the conjunctiva caused by four serovars of *Chlamydia trachomatis*. This organism is also responsible for a common reproductive tract infection, but the serovars that infect the genital tract usually do not infect the eye. Trachoma is the major infectious and preventable cause of blindness. Of all causes of blindness, it is second after cataract. Trachoma generally occurs where there is poverty, poor hygiene, and poor access to water. It is a disease of families; if one sibling is infected, more than 50% of others are likely to be infected with or without clinical signs. Blindness occurs after repeated infections and is 2–3 times more common in women than in men.

2. Current global burden and rating within the overall burden of disease

It is estimated that trachoma affects 146 million persons, and 500 million are at risk of the disease. An estimated 5.9 million people are blind or are at immediate risk for trachoma-associated blindness. Trachoma accounts for 15.5% of the global burden of blindness.

3. Feasibility (biological) of elimination/eradication

Elimination of blinding trachoma is possible, but eradication of *C. trachomatis* seems impossible. Trachoma has disappeared from North America and Europe because of improved socioeconomic conditions and hygiene.

4. Estimated costs and benefits of elimination/eradication

Both surgical and nonsurgical interventions for trachoma control are highly cost-effective. Evans &

Ransom employ a new measure — handicap-adjusted life years (HALYs) — a composite of years lost from both morbidity and mortality. During the 30 years of a trachoma control programme, the costs were US$ 11 per HALY saved for nonsurgical intervention and US$ 59 per HALY saved for surgical intervention.

5. Key strategies to accomplish the objectives

A new strategy (SAFE) has been developed from past knowledge and new techniques based on recent epidemiologic and control studies, as outlined below.

S: Surgery to correct lid deformity and prevent blindness. A simple tarsal rotation technique can be performed by eye nurses in 10 minutes.
A: Antibiotics for acute infections and/or community control — tetracycline ointment twice a day for 6 weeks or the new macrolide antibiotic, azithromycin, in a single dose. Operational research is required to work out the best regimen.
F: Facial hygiene. Clean faces are associated with a lower prevalence of trachoma. Behavioural change can be introduced and sustained even in poor areas with little water.
E: Environmental change — improved access to water and sanitation and health education.

   Because SAFE depends on community development/good public health practice, it involves not only the ministry of health but ministries of agriculture and water and sanitation. Beyond medical intervention, health education and community involvement are central to the success of this strategy.

   In addition to SAFE, a new simplified grading scheme has been developed for detecting and grading active infection in communities:

TF: follicular disease (the presence of five or more follicles in the upper tarsal conjunctiva);
TI: intense inflammation (pronounced inflammatory thickening of the upper tarsal conjunctiva that obscures more than half of the normal deep tarsal vessels);
TS: trachomatous scarring (the presence of scarring in the tarsal conjunctiva);
TT: trachomatous trichiasis (at least one eyelash rubs on the eyeball);

* Contributed by Joseph A. Cook, Program for Tropical Disease Research, The Edna McConnell Clark Foundation, New York, NY, USA

CO: corneal opacity (easily visible corneal opacity over the pupil).

WHO has organized an Alliance for Global Elimination of Trachoma by the Year 2020 (GET 2020), including nongovernmental organizations concerned with blindness prevention (Christoffel Blinded Mission, International Eye Foundation, Sight Savers International, Helen Keller International, Swiss Red Cross, The Carter Center, WorldVision, etc.), foundations (Edna McConnell Clark, Hilton, and Gulbenkian), bilateral agencies (such as DANIDA), and the private sector (Pfizer Inc.)

6. Research needs

In the absence of a vaccine, operational research with regard to the SAFE strategy is needed for the following: testing and validation of rapid community assessment techniques; azithromycin regimens; cost-benefit studies; surveillance/monitoring studies; and barriers to the acceptance of the preventive surgical procedure.

7. Status of elimination/eradication efforts to date

Trachoma decreases and even disappears with improved economic and social conditions and is absent from North America and Europe. Morocco has embarked on a plan to eliminate trachoma from five southern provinces in a programme supported by WHO, the Edna McConnell Clark Foundation, Pfizer Inc., and the World Bank. Pfizer is donating azithromycin to the programme and supporting efforts to advance health education and community participation.

8. Principal challenges to elimination/eradication

The principal challenge is generating awareness of both the problem within countries and the feasibility of control. The relative simplicity and low technological requirements of the strategy make trachoma elimination feasible, even in the poorest countries where it remains a public health problem.

Tuberculosis*

1. Brief description of the condition/disease

Tuberculosis (TB) is a bacterial disease caused by organisms of the *Mycobacterium tuberculosis* complex (*M. tuberculosis, M. bovis,* and *M. africanum*). It is transmitted primarily by airborne droplets; infection occurs when susceptible persons inhale infectious droplets produced by the exhalations (coughs and sneezes) of persons with respiratory tract TB. The risk for infection is directly related to the duration and intensity of exposure to air contaminated with these droplets. Most HIV-negative infected persons react to the purified protein derivative (PPD) tuberculin skin test, and 5–10% of HIV-negatives will develop clinically apparent TB. Infection is more likely to progress to clinical disease in the presence of certain risk factors, including time since infection and level of cell-mediated immunity. Of known risk factors, HIV infection may be the most potent, with up to 50% of persons with TB/HIV co-infection developing TB.

TB can be diagnosed presumptively if acid-fast bacilli (AFB) are found in the sputum, body fluids, or tissue, or by a combination of clinical symptoms, chest radiograph abnormality, and positive PPD skin test. However, definitive diagnosis requires isolation and identification of organisms of *M. tuberculosis* complex from a clinical specimen. Diagnosis of extrapulmonary TB is more difficult because it requires tissue biopsy or body fluids, which usually contain only a few organisms.

2. Current global burden and rating within the overall burden of disease

Throughout the world tuberculosis causes significant morbidity and mortality, with 2–3 million deaths annually and 8–10 million new cases (half of which are infectious AFB smear-positive pulmonary TB). Moreover, tuberculosis has infected 1–2000 million persons who are at risk of developing active disease.

Untreated, it is fatal in up to 50% of cases. However, effective chemotherapy has significantly reduced morbidity and mortality.

In developed countries, TB morbidity has decreased to low levels. In most developing countries, it remains one of the most common causes of morbidity and mortality. The World Bank estimates that over 25% of avoidable adult deaths worldwide are caused by TB. In many countries, case rates have not changed appreciably during the past several decades, and in areas where HIV infection is common, TB cases have increased dramatically.

3. Feasibility (biological) of elimination/eradication

Control measures are the same for developed and developing countries. However, the quality of these measures and the degree of their application differ greatly.

There are four general strategies for controlling tuberculosis:

• The most important and universally applied strategy is the early identification and treatment of persons with infectious TB. This strategy cures the affected person *and* renders the patient non-infectious within a few weeks, thus interrupting transmission in the community.

• Identification and treatment of persons with non-infectious TB (e.g. extrapulmonary TB, culture-negative pulmonary TB, primary TB in children, and TB infection without active disease) prevents infectious cases and subsequent TB transmission.

• Use of BCG vaccine which is commonly given to infants and children in developing countries. The vaccine is less commonly used in developed countries. Although BCG vaccine does protect young children against serious and fatal forms of TB, it does not reliably prevent the development of adult pulmonary TB. Consequently, it has no epidemiological impact on transmission of the disease.

Elimination of TB is feasible for the reasons outlined below.

• Infectious TB is relatively easy to identify by AFB smear. TB is treatable and curable, with cure rates approaching 100% when modern short-course therapy is used, and highly effective regimens costing as little as US$ 18 are available. Early diagnosis and

* Contributed by Bess Miller and Carl Schieffelbein, Division of Tuberculosis Elimination, Centers for Disease Control and Elimination, Atlanta, GA, USA.

effective treatment significantly reduce transmission. An excellent example of the effect of case-finding and treatment on reducing TB transmission was the U.S. Public Health Service (PHS) programme in Alaska where the annual infection rates in young children decreased from 25% to 1% between 1950 and 1960. The provision of short-course therapy with direct supervision to ensure cure is the cornerstone of the WHO "DOTS" (directly observed treatment–short course) strategy.

• Infected persons at increased risk of developing infectious TB can be identified through tuberculin screening of high-risk populations. TB is preventable by the administration of isoniazid preventive therapy (chemoprophylaxis) to those at risk of developing the disease. The efficacy of preventive therapy has been adequately demonstrated by clinical trials conducted by the PHS. More recent studies in developing countries have also found isoniazid-preventive therapy to be effective in HIV-infected persons.

• Humans are the primary reservoir of TB. Except for dairy cattle infected by *M. bovis*, no other important animal or environmental reservoirs of infection exists. In developed countries, testing of dairy herds and slaughter of infected animals and pasteurization of milk have virtually eliminated this problem. Moreover, in developing countries where *M. bovis* disease in cattle remains endemic, human disease associated with *M. bovis* does not appear to be common.

• In developed countries, TB has retreated into focal pockets that can be targeted for intensified control efforts. However, eliminating TB in these countries depends in part on global elimination because of imported cases. Although improved screening and prevention programmes targeting immigrants from countries with high TB rates will reduce the number of imported cases, tuberculosis in foreign-born persons will continue to occur until TB is eliminated globally.

• The World Bank has shown that short-course TB therapy is one of the most cost-effective health interventions available, comparing favourably with measles immunization, oral rehydration, and HIV screening of blood donors.

4. Estimated costs and benefits of elimination/eradication

No accurate costs for global elimination of TB are available. The immediate global task is to control

TB. Clearly, for a condition causing 8 million cases and 3 million deaths each year, the costs of disease and temporary disability are enormous. WHO has reported that TB treatment is a very cost-effective intervention, and DOTS is the key treatment strategy. However, WHO estimates that only about 30% of persons with TB worldwide have access to DOTS. Controlling TB in HIV-positive persons will ease the burden on general health services providing care for people with HIV/AIDS and their families and will add to the period of healthy life for people with HIV/AIDS.

WHO-estimates that to implement the DOTS strategy in India for 30% of the population will cost US$ 98.6 million. Global control of TB, leading to elimination, will cost over US$ 500 million and require many decades of sustained effort.

5. Key strategies to accomplish the objective

The DOTS strategy must be expanded and sustained where it is working well, and made easier to implement in both vertical and horizontal health-care delivery systems. In addition, more efficient methods to ensure the provision of curative treatment need to be identified and tried in demonstration projects.

6. Research needs

• The greatest need is for a new, safe, and effective vaccine to prevent the development of TB in already infected persons. Without such a vaccine, global TB elimination will not be realistic. Recent research has produced several types of candidate vaccines that are effective in animal models; clinical (human) trials of one or more vaccines are anticipated within the next several years. According to WHO, a new vaccine for TB will take 15 years to develop, given the most optimistic scenario.

• An inexpensive, rapid, accurate, and easily applied test is needed for diagnosing TB infection and disease. The ideal tests would be more sensitive and easier to perform than the tuberculin skin test and AFB microscopy.

• Research is also needed in the following areas: further shortening of TB therapy, especially with more widely spaced dosing that could be supervised, to improve the outcome of treatment (several promising new drugs are in various stages of investigation); improved methods to identify infected persons at risk of developing TB (this will permit targeting of preventive therapy to those who will benefit the most); alternatives to isoniazid preventive therapy which are shorter, safer, and better accepted; operational research into how to make delivery services more effective; and rapid transfer into practice of new technologies, which must be cost-effective even in poor countries.

7. Status of elimination/eradication efforts to date

Better use of current tools and implementation of new tools are necessary to control TB globally. WHO reports that many cases remain undiagnosed and receive no or inadequate treatment. These patients commonly are persistently infectious, chronically ill, more likely to die, and often carry drug-resistant strains. WHO estimates that if established "targets for case detection and cure could be met by the year 2000, we can expect to avert 70 million cases and 30 million deaths over the next 20 years." "Every year of delay in reaching targets will

be responsible for approximately 2.2 million extra cases and one million extra deaths . . ."

Unfortunately, widespread implementation of the WHO DOTS strategy is proceeding slowly. Current WHO estimates are that only 25% of TB patients in developing countries have access to DOTS services.

8. Principal challenges to elimination/eradication

The following are challenges to TB elimination: obtaining and continuing the political will of governments to support a strong TB-control effort; obtaining and continuing funding assistance for poor countries where most of the TB epidemic is occurring; assuring an ongoing drug supply; demonstrating the good return that investing in TB control and prevention programmes provides; evaluating programmes for successes; and a global strategic plan that would help ensure identification of funding priorities and present a concerted approach to the prevention, control, and eventual elimination of tuberculosis as a public health problem.

3. Parasitic diseases

Chagas disease or American trypanosomiasis*

1. Brief description of the condition/disease

Chagas disease, also known as American trypanosomiasis, is caused by the parasitic protozoan *Trypanosoma cruzi* and is transmitted primarily by triatomine insects; it can also be transmitted by blood transfusion. Neither an effective vaccine nor therapy is available. In approximately 30% of cases, chronic, often severe and life-threatening cardiac or digestive tract disease occurs 20–30 years after initial infection.

2. Current global burden and rating within the overall burden of disease

The disease is believed to affect 16–18 million people, primarily in Central and South America; an estimated 100 million people are at risk, accounting for approximately 25% of the entire population of this region. Chagas disease accounts for an estimated 45 000 deaths each year and is ranked third behind malaria and schistosomiasis by WHO in terms of global burden as a tropical disease.

3. Feasibility (biological) of elimination/eradication

WHO has targeted elimination of domestic transmission of Chagas disease. Because it exists as a zoonosis, complete eradication is not feasible; however, control of human transmission is considered achievable by eliminating domestic insect vector populations.

4. Estimated costs and benefits of elimination/eradication

Early estimates suggested that effective control could result in medical and economic benefits ex-

ceeding US$ 53 million per year, in the Sonthern Cone conutries alone, compared with an estimated total cost of US$ 190–350 million for the 10-year programme. More recent (1997) estimates suggest that the overall benefits of disease elimination could exceed US$ 3500 million per year.

5. Key strategies to accomplish the objective(s)

Elimination efforts focus on domiciliary insecticide applications using residual pyrethroids, improvement of housing conditions, and blood bank surveillance.

6. Research needs

Research needs include studies of vector population biology and genetics, evaluation of the impact of current vector-control programmes, tools for more effective blood bank screening, new effective drugs for treatment, and studies on immunopathogenesis.

7. Status of elimination/eradication efforts to date

Through the efforts of the Southern Cone Initiative, the chief regional vector *Triatoma infestans* has been virtually eliminated from most of Uruguay and Chile, from much of its original distribution in Brazil and Argentina, and from regions of Paraguay and southern Bolivia, resulting in effective interruption of disease transmission in these countries. A 70% reduction of incidence of *T. cruzi* infection in young age groups has been achieved between 1985 and 1997.

8. Principal challenges to elimination/eradication

Effective coordination, thoroughness, and long-term sustainability of vector control efforts are the primary challenges to elimination efforts.

* Contributed by C. Ben Beard, Centers for Disease Control and Prevention, Atlanta, GA, USA; and Chris J. Schofield, London School of Hygiene and Tropical Medicine, London, England, the ECLAT network, and World Health Organization, Geneva, Switzerland.

Lymphatic filariasis*

1. Brief description of the condition/disease

Lymphatic filariasis is a tropical disease caused by the parasitic worms *Wuchereria bancrofti* or *Brugia malayi*. Infection with these parasites leads to a variety of clinical manifestations, including lymphoedema and elephantiasis of the leg, genital disease (including hydrocele, chylocele, and elephantiasis of the scrotum and penis) and recurrent acute secondary bacterial infections, commonly known as "acute attacks". The majority of infected persons are asymptomatic, but virtually all have subclinical lymphatic damage, and approximately 40% have renal involvement (proteinuria and haematuria). Tropical pulmonary eosinophilia, a rare progressive lung disease, is caused by inflammatory reactions against the parasite in the lungs.

When an infected mosquito takes a blood meal, the larval form of the parasite enters the skin, migrates to the lymphatic vessels, and develops over 6–12 months into adult worms, which cause damage and dilatation of the lymphatic vessels. Fertile adult females, during their 4–6 year life span, release millions of microfilariae into the blood, which are taken up by mosquitos; further development inside the mosquito is required before the parasite larva is again infectious for humans.

2. Current global burden and rating within the overall burden of disease

Although lymphatic filariasis infrequently causes death, it is a major cause of clinical morbidity and disability. WHO ranks lymphatic filariasis as the second leading cause of disability worldwide. The economic burden of the disease is poorly defined, but the costs to India alone are estimated at US$ 1500 million. In 1990, the estimated burden of disease was 850 000 disability-adjusted life years (DALYs).

Approximately 120 million persons in tropical areas of the world are actually infected with the parasite, but those at-risk are estimated at 1100 million. Of these infections, 90% are caused by *W. bancrofti*; *B. malayi* (10%) is limited to Asia and parts of the South Pacific. An estimated 25 million men suffer from genital disease (most commonly

hydrocele); an estimated 15 million persons, the majority of whom are women, have lymphoedema or elephantiasis of the leg. The devastating social and psychological impact of these disfiguring conditions is only beginning to be understood.

3. Feasibility (biological) of elimination/eradication

The International Task Force for Disease Eradication considers lymphatic filariasis to be one of only six "eradicable or potentially eradicable" diseases. Factors favouring eradication include inefficient transmission (several hundred infective mosquito bites are required to produce a fertile adult worm pair) and, at least for *W. bancrofti*, the absence of a nonhuman reservoir. Because new drugs and drug combinations are now available that profoundly suppress microfilaria levels in the blood for ≥12 months after a single dose, elimination is possible with annual single-dose mass treatment. In 1997, the World Health Assembly called for global elimination of lymphatic filariasis as a public health problem. Lymphatic filariasis has already been eliminated from several countries, both as a result of targeted programmes (e.g. Japan and parts of China) and improved sanitation (e.g. the USA where *W. bancrofti* was endemic in South Carolina until the 1930s).

4. Estimated costs and benefits of elimination/eradication

Annual costs for mass treatment with available drug combinations are approximately US$ 0.05–0.10 per person. These efforts may have to be sustained for 5 years or longer to assure interruption of transmission. Benefits would include prevention of tremendous social and psychological suffering from chronic disease and improved economic productivity. If the estimated costs of lymphatic filariasis in India (US$ 1500 million) are similar to those in the rest of the world, the global economic benefit of lymphatic filariasis elimination could approach $4000 million per year.

5. Key strategies to accomplish the objectives

Global elimination of lymphatic filariasis means interrupting transmission of infection, and reducing

---

* Contributed by David Addiss, Centers for Disease Control and Prevention, Atlanta, GA, USA.

the suffering of persons with chronic disease, including appropriate treatment of lymphoedema and elephantiasis. The main strategy recommended for interruption of transmission is annual mass treatment of at-risk populations in endemic areas with single doses of albendazole in combination with either ivermectin or DEC; ancillary vector control can be helpful but is not required. To alleviate the suffering, the principal strategy is health education and training so that affected individuals learn the importance of scrupulous hygiene and other measures and the techniques necessary to achieve them.

6. Research needs

Diagnostic and therapeutic tools are already available for global elimination of lymphatic filariasis. Additional research is needed to identify and evaluate techniques for rapid assessment and mapping of the disease, to develop mechanisms for surveillance and for monitoring the effectiveness of interventions, to identify optimal drug-delivery systems, and to assess the cost-effectiveness of intervention strategies. Research is also needed to optimize the effectiveness of drugs and drug combinations in killing the adult stage of the parasite.

7. Status of elimination/eradication efforts to date

Recognizing the availability of these new tools and a proven strategy for using them, the World Health Assembly in 1997 defined an international political will for this initiative by resolving to eliminate lymphatic filariasis as a public health problem globally. By November 1997, 13 countries in Asia, South America, and Africa had announced national plans for elimination of lymphatic filariasis, and seven of these countries had already begun implementing these plans. For example, in India alone, 40 million people have been targeted to receive a single dose of DEC on "National Filariasis Day."

8. Principal challenges to elimination/eradication

Challenges include: developing and sustaining the global, regional, and national will required for filariasis elimination; and developing accurate and efficient methods to certify elimination.

Onchocerciasis*

1. Brief description of the condition/disease

Onchocerca volvulus infection (i.e. "river blind-ness"), which is caused by filariid parasites that are long-lived (8–15 years), is characterized by chronic skin and eye lesions. It is transmitted by *Simulium* blackflies that breed in rapidly flowing rivers and streams. The embryonic stage (microfilaria), re-leased by female worms, causes most of the pathol-ogy. Human infection occurs from the bite of a blackfly that harbours one or more infectious (third-stage) *O. volvulus* larvae. Male and female worms gather in groups of five or six, intertwined and en-cased in a fibrous capsule that forms a palpable nod-ule. The female worms produce thousands of microfilariae (each about the size of a period on this page), which leave the nodule and migrate into the host's skin, eyes, and other organs. Persons with many fertilized female worms can harbour as many as 200 million microfilariae. The microfilariae live for 9–18 months but cannot develop into adult worms without first passing through the *Simulium* blackfly vector. In these insects, the microfilariae transform in the course of 6–12 days into the third-stage larvae that are infective to humans. There is no known animal reservoir for *O. volvulus*.

Several aspects of this life-cycle affect potential eradicability. First, only the few microfilariae that succeed in passing through both human and blackfly hosts reach adulthood. Second, the blackfly must bite at least twice to transmit the infection: once to acquire microfilariae from an infected person, and again to transmit the infectious larvae to another person. Finally, rarely do more than 5% of blackflies harbour infectious larvae at a given time, and most of these flies have only one or two such larvae ready to inoculate. Therefore, the transmission cycle has only one point of amplification (through humans) and is relatively susceptible to interruption.

* Contributed by Frank O Richards, Centers for Disease Control and Prevention Atlanta, GA, USA; Emanuel Miri, The Carter Center of Emory University, Atlanta, GA, USA; Stefanie Meredith, Task Force for Child Survival and Development, CDC, Atlanta, GA, USA; Ronald Guderian, (formerly) Ecuador Onchocerciasis Con-trol Program, Seattle, WA, USA; Mauricio Sauerbrey, Oncho-cerciasis Elimination Program of the Americas, Guatemala; Hans Remme, Tropical Disease Research Programme, WHO, Geneva, Switzerland; Randall Packard, Emory University Rollins School of Public Health, Atlanta, GA, USA; Jean-Michel Ndiaye, Africa Re-gional Advisor in Health/Guinea-worm, UNICEF, Abidjan, Côte d'Ivoire.

2. Current global burden and rating within the overall burden of disease

Onchocerciasis is known to be endemic in 37 coun-tries. In 1995, the WHO Expert Committee on Onchocerciasis estimated that 123 million persons were at risk of contracting the disease, and 17–18 million were infected, of whom about 270000 were blind and another 500000 severely visually impaired. About 95% of infected persons reside in Africa, where the disease is most severe along the major rivers in 30 countries in a belt spanning the northern and central part of the continent. Outside Africa, onchocerciasis occurs in Mexico, Guatemala, Ecua-dor, Colombia, Venezuela, and Brazil in the Ameri-cas, and in Yemen in Asia.

3. Feasibility (biological) of elimination/eradication

In 1993, the International Task Force for Disease Elimination did not list onchocerciasis as one of the six diseases suitable for eradication. However, onchocerciasis was listed as a disease, one aspect of which (blindness) could be eliminated. The difficul-ties in eradication include: the long life-span of the adult worms: the occurrence of reinfections; and lack of vaccines and acceptable drugs to kill the adult worms (macrofilaricide).

However, reconsideration of these difficulties is now appropriate, given the considerable progress made towards elimination of all morbidity from onchocerciasis in the Onchocerciasis Control Pro-gramme (OCP) areas in West Africa and in the Americas. Using vector control, the OCP has been very successful in interrupting transmission of this disease. After 20 years, onchocerciasis is no longer a public health problem in the original OCP area. Whereas infection rates in the programme's most severely affected country, Burkina Faso, were 80–90% when the programme began, the highest rates in 1995 were <2%. All 30 million persons at risk in the 11 countries of the OCP are being protected, and 125000 to 200000 have been prevented from becom-ing blind. About 10 million children born since the programme began are free from onchocerciasis, and 25 million hectares of land — enough to support 17 million persons — along West African rivers are now available for resettlement. In the Americas, data strongly suggest that semiannual mass distribution of ivermectin, without vector control, has interrupted transmission in 7 of 14 known foci, including those in Colombia and Ecuador, where one of the most efficient vectors in the world (*Simulium exiguum*) exists. If transmission can be interrupted with a free and easily deliverable medicine, the disease could potentially be eradicable. Furthermore, computer models and observations suggest that repeated ivermectin treatment might affect the fecundity of adult females or longevity of adult males, thus reducing the duration of mass treatment programmes to less than the life span of the adult parasites (8–15 years). Nongovernmental development organizations (NGDOs), bilateral and multilateral institutions, and national governments are providing the international momentum behind major programmes, and industry (Merck & Co.) is donating the drug. Finally, the problem is, unlike lymphatic filariasis, restricted to rural Africa and Latin America. Thus, onchocerciasis may now be eligible to be included on the list of diseases for potential eradication.

4. Estimated costs and benefits of elimination/eradication

In African communities with severe (hyperendemic) onchocerciasis of the savanna type, 15% of the population can be blind and up to 40% of adults can be visually impaired. Visual impairment is a major occupational and social obstacle and reduces the life span of affected persons by an average of 10 years. Agricultural production decreases, young children are forced to care for their parents, and adolescents emigrate because of the fear of becoming blind. Ultimately, the village is further impoverished or completely abandoned. In areas where blinding onchocerciasis is rare, onchocercal skin disease occurs in up to 30% of the population; 8 million persons suffer from troublesome itching associated with dermal onchocerciasis, making it difficult for them to work, study, or interact socially. The unsightly skin changes may result in poor self-esteem and social ostracism. Intensive research is under way on the economic impact of onchocercal skin disease.

5. Key strategies to accomplish the objectives

The OCP, which began in seven countries in 1974, used a strategy of interrupting transmission via vector control. The programme comprised aerial larviciding, supplemented by ground and water-based handspraying of blackfly breeding sites in rivers over a vast area of West Africa. In 1986, operations were extended to parts of four other countries to prevent reinvasion of the core area by blackflies. Replication of the OCP was not practical for 87% of the onchocerciasis-affected population living outside the OCP area.

In 1987, the introduction of ivermectin (Mectizan) resulted in a new strategy that enabled assistance to be extended to other populations. The drug kills *Onchocerca* microfilariae with almost no serious side-effects, and its effects after one oral dose last for approximately a year. In 1987, Merck & Co. announced its decision to provide the drug without cost in whatever quantities were needed and for as long as necessary to treat and prevent onchocerciasis. Merck also established an independent group of international scientists, the Mectizan Expert Committee, to evaluate applications for supplies of the drug.

The donation by Merck & Co. prompted national and international health workers in the affected countries to develop systems capable of distributing the orally administered drug once or twice a year to persons in remote villages. Many programmes for community-based distribution of Mectizan are assisted by NGDOs, which have demonstrated their flexibility, creativity, and rapid response to the challenge. The NGDOs have used delivery of what has become a popular drug in the communities as an entry point for developing broader health care services. A 10-member NGDO coalition has been established internationally, and national coalitions of NGDOs have been established in some countries.

In December 1995 the World Bank, encouraged by these successes, launched another regional programme — the African Programme for Onchocerciasis Control (APOC) — for the remaining areas of Africa. The primary goal of APOC is to eliminate onchocerciasis as a public health problem in these areas of Africa by the year 2007 by reaching the remaining 50–60 million persons at risk of potentially blinding onchocerciasis and/or severe skin disease. Unlike the OCP, APOC will use annual community-based distribution of Mectizan as its primary control strategy. Similarly, the Onchocerciasis Elimination Program for the Americas (OEPA), established after a Pan American Health Organization resolution in 1991 and aided by the InterAmerican Development Bank, also aims to eliminate onchocerciasis as a public health problem in the Americas by 2007 through Mectizan delivery. On both continents, the strategy entails rapidly determining the severity and distribution of onchocerciasis in remote areas and communities by testing a carefully selected sample of the populations and communities using new microcomputer-based mapping techniques and noninvasive, field-based diagnostic methods. Rapid-assessment field techniques are based on classification of communities by the prevalence of nodules (hyperendemicity is generally defined as rates ≥40%). Once the "at-risk" communities are identified, Mectizan is offered annually (or in some countries in the Americas, biannually) for an indefinite period to all healthy persons except mothers who are nursing <1-week-old infants.

6. Research needs

Research is needed concerning the following: mechanisms of surveillance; GIS (geographic information system) applications; computer-modelling of transmission of the parasite; PCR/DNA probes for infective larvae in blackflies; impact of prolonged ivermectin treatment on onchocercal skin disease; adult worm longevity/fecundity (through antigen detection techniques); monitoring of transmission; aspects of sustainability; economic impact; development of new macrofilaricides; and adapting the programme (without disrupting the current momentum) to other suitable drugs that can be used at the community level to control or eradicate other widespread diseases, such as combination therapy for lymphatic filariasis or praziquantel for schistosomiasis.

7. Status of elimination/eradication efforts

The progressive increase in the numbers treated with ivermectin has been impressive — from 500000 persons in 1988 to >20 million in 1997. The World Bank signed a declaration of intent to reach the remaining 50–60 million persons at risk of potentially blinding onchocerciasis and/or severe skin disease and eliminate onchocerciasis as a public health problem in Africa by 2007. Similarly, the Onchocerciasis Elimination Program for the Americas aims to eliminate onchocerciasis as a public problem in the Americas by 2007. More than 95% of known hyperendemic communities in the Americas are under treatment. Merck & Co. will provide 410 million tablets of Mectizan, valued at several hundred million US$, during the initiative; over 100-million doses of Mectizan have safely been given since the donation began in 1987.

8. Principal challenges to elimination/eradication

Challenges to elimination include the following: adequate funding; establishment by APOC and OEPA of effective and lasting partnerships with the coalition participants; continued refinement of the model of sustainable community-based distribution of Mectizan to control onchocerciasis; surveillance mechanisms for "sustainabilty"; management training at the ministry of health level; development of new macrofilaricides; difficulties associated with importing the drug; the relatively short shelf-life (2 years) of ivermectin; and certification criteria that are internationally accepted for elimination of morbidity and transmission.

Schistosomiasis*

1. Brief description of the condition/disease

Schistosomiasis is a tropical disease caused by several species of parasitic worms of the genus *Schistosoma* that live within human blood vessels. The female worm produces eggs that are fertilized by male worms and deposited in the vessel walls. The eggs either leave the body in the faeces or urine, or remain in the tissues where they cause inflammation and scarring. Symptoms are related to the location and number of eggs. *S. mansoni* and *S. japonicum* primarily cause disease of the intestines and liver, including diarrhoea, abdominal pain, fibrosis of the liver and collateral circulation. *S. haematobium* primarily affects the bladder and urogenital system, causing bloody urine and problems with micturition and fertility. If the eggs reach fresh water, they hatch, and the embryo (miracidium) swims in search of a susceptible intermediate host (snail species). Within the snail, they develop into larvae (cercariae) which are shed into the water and then become infective for humans.

Infection occurs when human skin contacts these fresh-water cercariae, which penetrate the skin, develop into adult worms, and migrate to the veins of the abdominal cavity, where the adult females release millions of eggs. The eggs escape to the lumen of the urinary bladder or intestine and are passed out during micturition or defecation, reach fresh water, and hatch into miracidia which infect the host snails that produce cercariae, and begin new infections.

2. Current global burden and rating within the overall burden of disease

An estimated 200 million persons in tropical areas of the world are infected with the parasites. Of these, 120 million persons are symptomatic and 20 million have severe disease, with manifestations that include hepatosplenomegaly and portal hypertension for intestinal schistosomiasis. For urinary schistosomiasis the disease manifestations range from haematuria to squamous cell cancer of the bladder. The loss in productivity resulting from schistosomiasis is 4–44 person-days per year.

* Contributed by Daniel G. Colley and David Addiss, Centers for Disease Control and Prevention, Atlanta, GA, USA; and Lester Chitsulo, CTD, World Health Organization, Geneva, Switzerland.

3. Feasibility (biological) of elimination/eradication

Humans are the principal reservoir of *S. mansoni* and *S. haematobium*. Although other mammals (e.g. baboons) can be permissive hosts and can be infected, they do not contribute significantly to human transmission in most endemic areas. Domestic and other animals can also be infected with *S. japonicum* and figure significantly in transmission where they share living areas or their faeces are used as fertilizer.

Comprehensive control programmes, including mass treatment with antischistosomal drugs, health education, application of molluscicides, and other measures have reduced the prevalence dramatically in many areas. However, although they often reduce morbidity and mortality, control programmes have not usually led to elimination or eradication of transmission. Examples of the exceptions, in which control programmes have eliminated transmission, include the lesser Antilles Islands of Antigua, Guadeloupe, Martinique, and St. Lucia. In Tunisia, no transmission has occurred since 1984. Schistosomiasis has been eradicated from Japan and Montserrat. Control interventions probably will stop transmission in Indonesia, Islamic Republic of Iran, Morocco, and Saudi Arabia during the next few years.

4. Estimated costs and benefits of elimination/eradication

Benefits of elimination include the following: potential earning of millions of dollars in tourism (e.g. in Malawi); savings in health expenditures for schistosomiasis; reduction in bladder cancer rates; decreases in premature death rates; and increases of approximately 4.5 million disability-adjusted life years worldwide.

5. Key strategies to accomplish the objective

A comprehensive approach to elimination is required. This would include mass treatment with praziquantel or other drugs; construction of wells and latrines; community health education to modify water use and sites of defecation/urination; and reduction of the vector snail populations through environmental modification and use of molluscicides.

6. Research needs

Research is needed in the following areas: vaccine development; simple field-applicable tools for diagnosis (e.g. a test for circulating antigen in urine or saliva); and continued search for drugs in case widespread resistance develops to praziquantel and oxamniquine.

7. Status of elimination/eradication efforts to date

Although control of schistosomiasis is considered a public health priority in many countries in which it is endemic, serious attempts at elimination/eradication have occurred in relatively few places. Antigua, Guadeloupe, Japan, Martinique, Montserrat, St Lucia, and Tunisia have conducted successful programmes. Large-scale control programmes in Brazil, Egypt, China, Indonesia (Sulawesi), Islamic Republic of Iran, Morocco, the Philippines, and Puerto Rico have achieved varying degrees of success in reducing prevalence and subsequent morbidity.

8. Principal challenges to elimination/eradication

Challenges include the need for effective treatment and retreatment delivery programmes; rapid, field-applicable tools to assess reinfection; comprehensive programmes, including provision and use of uncontaminated fresh water; a vaccine; and cost-effective methods for snail control. Elimination/eradication is not a feasible goal in sub-Saharan Africa where 80% of transmission is currently taking place and where effective morbidity control should be the aim of all Member States.

4. Viral diseases

Hepatitis B virus infection*

1. Brief description of the condition/disease

Hepatitis B virus (HBV) is transmitted through percutaneous or permucosal exposure to blood or body fluids, producing an acute or chronic infection. Most acute infections are asymptomatic. Fewer than 10% of children and 33% of adults have acute hepatitis B, which often results in hospitalization and — in approximately 0.1% of patients — in acute hepatic failure and death. HBV regularly produces chronic infection in infants (90%) and young children (30–60%) and, less frequently (1–6%), in older children, adolescents, and adults. Among adults, chronic HBV infection can cause death from chronic liver disease (CLD, e.g. cirrhosis) or primary hepatocellular carcinoma (PHC). The risk for a liver-disease-associated death among persons with chronic HBV infection is 25% for those who acquired infection as an infant or young child, and 15% for those who acquired infection as an adolescent or adult. HBV infection also can produce extrahepatic manifestations, including polyarteritis nodosa and membrano-proliferative glomerulonephritis.

The prevalence of chronic HBV infection varies worldwide; it is highly endemic (>8% prevalence) in Africa, the Pacific Islands, parts of South America, and most of Asia, as well as in ethnically defined populations in Australia, New Zealand, and the USA. The high prevalence of infection is sustained by transmission during the perinatal period and early childhood. In populations with intermediate endemicity (2–8% prevalence), perinatal and early childhood transmission accounts for most HBV infection. Endemicity is low (<2% prevalence) in Australia, New Zealand, Western Europe, and the USA. Most acute infections occur among adolescents and adults, but perinatal and early childhood infections contribute substantially to the prevalence of chronic infection, and populations in which HBV infection is highly endemic may reside in these areas.

2. Current burden and rating within the overall burden of disease

Estimates derived from regional data on prevalence of infection in the general population indicate that 360 million people worldwide have chronic HBV infection: 78% in Asia; 16% in Africa; 3% in South America; and 3% in Europe, North America and Oceania combined. Of these 360 million HBV-infected people, 55–92 million (15–25%) are expected to die at 45–55 years of age from HBV-related CLD. An estimated 1 million people die annually from HBV-related CLD or PHC. Although etiology-specific death rates for CLD are not available in most countries, CLD or PHC is among the five leading causes of death among adults in many developing countries. In countries in which HBV infection is highly endemic, most CLD is HBV-related; in countries in which endemicity is low, such as the USA, 10–15% of CLD is HBV-related.

3. Feasibility (biological) of elimination/eradication

Immunization with plasma-derived or recombinant hepatitis B vaccine confers a high level of protection against acute and chronic infection. Pre-exposure vaccination prevents >95% of infections, and postexposure vaccination of infants at risk for perinatal infection prevents 90–95% of infections. The initial vaccination series confers protection against chronic infection for at least 15 years, and HBV transmission has been eliminated in populations 10 years after introduction of routine infant vaccination. Most chronically infected persons remain so over their lifetime, but their potential infectivity decreases because of the decline in HBV titre (HB_eAg-positivity). The combined effects of immunization and declining infectivity make elimination of HBV infection feasible. Eradication of HBV infection requires sustained elimination of transmission over the number of years needed for persons with chronic infection to be no longer in the population. The increased use of effective antiviral

---

* Contributed by Harold S. Margolis, Centers for Disease Control and Prevention, Atlanta, GA, USA.

agents to treat chronic HBV infection could hasten its elimination.

Humans are the only known host for HBV. Although experimental infection can be produced in some great apes, they do not appear to be a reservoir. Variants of HBV have been described which appear resistant to vaccine-induced antibody. However, failure of pre-exposure vaccination caused by these variants has not been demonstrated.

4. Estimated costs and benefits of elimination/eradication

Economic analyses have shown routine infant vaccination to be cost-effective in preventing the acute and chronic sequelae of HBV infection in populations in which endemic HBV infection is high or low. In China (Province of Taiwan), the rate of chronic HBV infection and PHC deaths decreased among children within 10 years of a sustained infant hepatitis B vaccination programme. However, because the costs of HBV-related CLD will occur many years in the future, some analyses have not found vaccination to be cost-saving or cost-effective. The economic effects of vaccination programmes to eliminate HBV transmission in populations with differing rates of infection have not been examined.

5. Key strategies to accomplish the objectives

The basic strategy to eliminate HBV transmission is to integrate hepatitis B vaccine into the routine infant vaccination schedule in a manner that will prevent perinatal and early childhood infection. In populations in which endemic HBV infection is high or intermediate, this generally requires beginning routine vaccination at birth to prevent perinatal transmission. However, using maternal HB_sAg screening, any country with the appropriate infrastructure could identify infants who require post-exposure vaccination soon after birth and routinely vaccinate all other infants. In countries in which the endemicity of HBV infection is intermediate or low, routine infant vaccination will prevent transmission among adolescents and adults after several decades. Elimination of transmission can be accelerated through catch-up vaccination of young children, adolescents, and high-risk adults.

6. Research needs

Country-specific data are needed on HBV infection and the burden of HBV-related disease, development of combination childhood vaccines that include hepatitis B, continued studies to determine the long-term efficacy of infant immunization and the need for booster doses of vaccine, population-based studies of the effectiveness of various vaccination strategies, possible effects of antibody-resistant variants of HBV in elimination of transmission, and the potential for HBV circulation in susceptible animals.

7. Status of elimination/eradication efforts to date

The World Health Assembly has recommended that all countries integrate hepatitis B vaccine into childhood (infant or, where appropriate, adolescent) vaccination schedules by 1997. Thus far, approximately 95 countries have included or are in the process of including hepatitis B vaccine in their childhood vaccination schedules. Population-based evaluation projects (e.g. in China (Province of Taiwan), the Gambia, Shanghai, and Alaska) have been developed to evaluate the effectiveness of various vaccination strategies, and in some, transmission has been eliminated.

8. Principle challenges to elimination/eradication

HBV is the first chronic infection considered for elimination/eradication. The principle challenges are to eliminate transmission and to maintain elimination for many decades. The primary barrier to elimination of HBV transmission is the cost of hepatitis B vaccine, especially for developing countries. Although the vaccine became available in the early 1980s, the cost appears to be higher relative to other childhood vaccines because it is a new vaccine produced with new technology. Other barriers include lack of knowledge about the relation between chronic HBV infection, CLD, and PHC; lack of local information on the HBV-related disease burden; and continued perception that because HBV-related CLD and PHC occur among adults, prevention of HBV infection is not an appropriate childhood vaccination activity, especially in countries where the endemicity is low.

Measles*

1. Brief description of the condition/disease

Measles is an acute disease characterized by fever, cough, coryza, conjunctivitis, and an erythematous maculopapular rash caused by infection with the measles virus (an RNA virus classified as *Morbillivirus* in the *Paramyxoviridae* family). Complications such as otitis media, bronchopneumonia, croup, and diarrhoea occur more commonly in young children. Acute encephalitis occurs in approximately one in every 1000 cases. Subacute sclerosing panencephalitis develops rarely (about 1 per 100 000) several years after infection. Measles is more severe in malnourished children in whom it can cause haemorrhagic rash, protein-losing enteropathy, oral sores, diarrhoea with dehydration, and severe skin infections. In children who are borderline nourished, measles often precipitates acute kwashiorkor and exacerbates vitamin A deficiency leading to blindness. In the USA, 1–2 of every 1000 reported cases are fatal. Case-fatality rates in developing countries are 3–5% and can reach 30% in high-risk communities. Case-fatality rates are also high in immunocompromised children, including those with HIV infection and leukaemia; the characteristic rash sometimes does not develop in these patients.

2. Current global burden and rating within the overall burden of disease

The number of measles cases reported worldwide to WHO declined from 4.4 million in 1980 to 1.3 million in 1990 and 0.8 million in 1996. However, measles reporting is incomplete; the actual burden from measles in 1996 was an estimated 36.5 million cases and 1 million deaths. The *Global burden of disease* attributes 10% of mortality from all causes among children <5 years of age to measles; it is the eighth leading cause of death worldwide, representing 2.7% of disability-adjusted life years in 1990.

3. Feasibility (biological) of elimination/eradication

Although nonhuman primates can be infected with measles virus, humans are believed to be the only reservoir capable of sustaining transmission of the virus. Acquired immunity after illness is permanent. Live attenuated measles virus, when administered at the recommended ages, produces >85% immunity after one dose and >90% immunity after two doses; and vaccine-induced immunity is long-lasting. Widespread vaccination (mass campaigns and routine vaccination) has resulted in interruption of measles virus transmission in a number of settings (e.g. the Gambia in 1968–69, the English-speaking Caribbean islands, Cuba, Chile, and possibly other countries in Latin America in the 1990s, and the USA over short periods in 1993, 1995, and 1996). However, sustaining elimination in large populations or regions is difficult because of importations of measles virus from endemic areas, which is facilitated by the frequency of air travel. This experience suggests eradication of measles is technically feasible with existing vaccines but will require a coordinated global effort over a relatively short period of time.

4. Estimated costs and benefits of elimination/eradication

Measles vaccination is one of the most cost-beneficial public health interventions. A preliminary economic analysis performed by the Children's Vaccine Initiative estimated expenditure of US$ 1100 million in 1995 for treatment of measles disease, and US$ 480 million for implementing the existing vaccination programme. Accelerating measles control, particularly in areas of low vaccination coverage and high disease burden, will probably be highly cost-effective. Cost-benefit and cost-effectiveness analyses for global measles elimination/eradication are under way.

5. Key strategies to accomplish the objective

Measles transmission can be interrupted if high population immunity is achieved rapidly through mass vaccination campaigns and/or routine immunization services. The Pan American Health Organization (PAHO) measles-elimination strategies are as

* Contributed by Peter M. Strebel, Centers for Disease Control and Prevention, Atlanta, GA, USA.

follows: conduct a one-time "catch-up" vaccination campaign targeting all children aged 9 months to 14 years; achieve and maintain high routine vaccination coverage; conduct periodic "follow-up" campaigns targeting all children aged 1–4 years; and enhance surveillance for cases with laboratory confirmation of measles virus infection and virus isolation to enable molecular identification of the geographical origin of the virus.

6. Research needs

The following areas warrant further investigation and research: the importance of adults in sustaining measles transmission and strategies to prevent adult outbreaks; the effectiveness of PAHO-style elimination strategies in African settings with large urban slums and high HIV-infection rates; the interrelations between HIV infection (or other immuno-compromising conditions) and measles disease/vaccination; strategies to improve the safety and ease of administration of measles vaccine in mass campaigns; and monitoring the safety of measles vaccination.

7. Status of elimination/eradication efforts to date

In 1996, the estimated global coverage with one dose of measles vaccine was 81%. Nevertheless, nearly 1 million measles-related deaths occur each year, half of them in Africa. The countries of the Americas are committed to eliminate measles by the year 2000, and the Pacific Island nations are expected to make a similar commitment in the near future. The European Advisory Group on the Expanded Programme on Immunization has recommended that measles be eliminated from Europe by the year 2007. The Regional Committee of the Eastern Mediterranean has adopted an elimination target of 2010. China and several southern African countries have embarked on accelerated measles control/elimination approaches.

8. Principal challenges to elimination/eradication

Challenges include: perception in developed countries that measles is a minor disease of little consequence; lack of political and financial support; ease of importation of measles virus, particularly through air travel; and need to mobilize global resources and collaboration among partner organizations and focus these over a relatively short period of time (3–5 years).

Rubella and congenital rubella syndrome*

1. Brief description of the condition/disease

Rubella usually presents as a mild or asymptomatic infection in adults and children. However, rubella infection in pregnant women, especially during the first trimester, can result in miscarriage, stillbirth, or the constellation of birth defects known as congenital rubella syndrome (CRS). The most commonly described CRS anomalies include nerve deafness, cataracts, cardiac anomalies, and mental retardation.

2. Current global burden and rating with the overall burden of disease

The global burden of rubella and CRS is undefined. Rubella is endemic in most countries. In a survey conducted by WHO in 1995, 78 of 214 countries (36%) had a national policy of rubella vaccination. Analysis of published serosurveys in several developing countries indicated a wide range of serosusceptibility in reproductive-aged women. Thus, the potential for outbreaks of rubella and subsequent CRS exist. More than 20000 infants are born with CRS each year in the Americas in the absence of major epidemics. Globally, an estimated 236000 CRS cases occur every non-epidemic year in developing countries. In countries with endemic rubella in the prevaccine era, the rate of CRS was 1 per 1000 live births.

3. Feasibility (biological) of elimination/eradication

Use of the established criteria for feasibility of eradication by the International Task force for Disease Eradication indicates that rubella and CRS can be eradicated. Since the introduction of rubella vaccine in the USA in 1969, the incidences of rubella and CRS have decreased by 99%.

The following factors favour elimination/eradication of rubella/CRS: humans are the only reservoir for rubella; rubella vaccine is highly effective in preventing rubella and CRS, and a combination vaccine with measles exists; and because of this combination vaccine, rubella elimination/eradication can be combined with the already existing measles elimination/eradication efforts.

4. Estimated costs and benefits of elimination/eradication

Rubella and CRS prevention is cost-effective. In the USA in 1982, the estimated lifetime cost of caring for a child with CRS was over US$ 200000. A cost–benefit analysis for rubella vaccine in the USA conducted in 1992 demonstrated a ratio of 11.1:1 when considering direct and indirect costs.

5. Key strategies to accomplish the objectives

The key strategies for countries with no rubella/CRS surveillance or rubella vaccination programme include: establishment of surveillance for rubella and CRS; implementation of a national rubella vaccination programme, particularly ensuring high level protection of reproductive-aged women as a means of direct protection; and prompt outbreak-control measures.

Countries that have an established rubella and CRS surveillance system and national rubella vaccination programme should include maintenance of high vaccination levels in preschool- and school-aged children and young adults (particularly women of childbearing age); intensification of diagnosis of and surveillance for rubella and CRS; and prompt control of rubella outbreaks.

6. Research needs

Research needs include development of rapid and non-invasive laboratory tests for diagnosis of rubella/CRS; and determination of the serosusceptibility to rubella among reproductive-aged women in developing countries to monitor the impact of the rubella vaccination programmes.

7. Status of elimination/eradication efforts to date

The USA has targeted a goal of eliminating indigenous rubella and CRS by the year 2000. PAHO

---

* Contributed by Susan E. Reef, Centers for Disease Control and Prevention, Atlanta, GA, USA.

has determined it would be premature to establish a hemispheric goal of rubella elimination, but this could be a logical development as progress continues with measles elimination.

8. Principal challenges to elimination/eradication

Challenges include establishing rubella and CRS as a priority in many developing countries; depending on the vaccination strategy implemented in countries, 30–40 years may be required for eradication/elimination of CRS; and lack of financial resources in many countries to sustain a vaccination programme because of the added cost of the rubella component of the vaccine and the necessity to ensure protection in reproductive-aged women.

Yellow fever*

1. Brief description of the condition/disease

Yellow fever (YF) is a multisystem disease of variable severity characterized in most cases by an acute, prostrating, but self-limited generalized febrile illness and, in persons who have the severe form of the disease, by a combination of hepatitis, generalized haemorrhages, proteinuria and myocarditis, and death in 25–50% of cases. The mosquito-borne flaviviral infection occurs naturally only in South America and Africa. In South America, sylvatic YF leads to sporadic cases and small outbreaks. However, following reversal of the gains achieved during the hemispheric campaign to eradicate *Aedes aegypti*, the principal mosquito vector of urban YF, most tropical and subtropical urban areas of the Americas are now at greater risk of urban epidemics than at any time in the last 50 years. In sub-Saharan Africa YF is a major public health problem occurring in an endemic pattern, with periodic urban epidemics due to interhuman transmission by *A. aegypti*. With extensive and rapid international air travel, the occurrence of YF outbreaks in either of these regions also increases the risk of introducing the virus into urban areas of the Pacific and Asia, where *A. aegypti* is also widespread.

2. Current global burden and rating within the overall burden of disease

Over the period 1986–95, 21 717 cases (5119 fatal) from Africa and 2018 cases (1301 fatal) from South America were reported to WHO, giving an annual average of 2000 and 200 cases, respectively. However, in specific studies, official reports of epidemics have underestimated incidence by factors ranging from 3- to 250-fold. Yellow fever was not included in the recent Global Burden of Disease and Injury Series; however, its reported incidence in sub-Saharan Africa is similar to that of reported *Neisseria meningitidis* episodes in that region.

3. Feasibility (biological) of elimination/eradication

Previous national and regional vaccination and *A. aegypti* eradication programmes have shown the feasibility of significantly reducing or eliminating disease transmission in areas where coverage with the attenuated vaccine was high or the mosquitos were eliminated in urban areas. Over a 15-year period when the vaccine was used consistently in French-speaking Africa, no outbreaks occurred even though epidemic transmission continued in neighbouring English-speaking countries. Although YF can never be eradicated because the virus is maintained in natural animal reservoirs human disease can be effectively eliminated by vaccination with the proven 17D vaccine, or in urban areas, by mosquito control.

4. Estimated costs and benefits of elimination/eradication

The estimated cost-effectiveness of YF vaccination in Nigeria is US$ 381–763 per case prevented and US$ 1904–3817 per death averted, depending on whether the vaccine was administered during emergency interventions or routinely (under EPI), respectively.

5. Key strategies to accomplish the objectives

While YF vaccine has recently been administered principally in *ad hoc* campaigns to contain outbreaks, the above cost-effectiveness analysis showed that routine administration under the EPI was sevenfold more efficient in preventing cases and deaths. In 1988, WHO and UNICEF recommended routine childhood and catch-up YF vaccination in Africa, but coverage rates typically range from <1% to 50%. A committed effort by national governments and international agencies to improve and maintain vaccination coverage is needed; administration at the same time as measles vaccine is a strategy to reduce administration costs and to link YF vaccine with a disease that has greater visibility. *A. aegypti* eradication is not considered feasible in all areas where the disease is endemic. Recent YF cases in unvaccinated Americans and Europeans visiting areas with endemic transmission underscore the underutilization of the vaccine by travellers.

* Contributed by Theodore F. Tsai, Centers for Disease Control and Prevention, Atlanta, GA, USA.

6. Research needs

High HIV infection rates overlap areas of Africa where universal YF vaccination is recommended. However, the vaccine's safety in HIV-infected persons remains unresolved. YF vaccine is safe in adults but carries a poorly studied potential for neurological side-effects in infants. Although vaccination is recommended at 9–12 months, the rate of serious neurological side-effects in that age group is unknown. Research is needed to improve vector surveillance methods and to develop practical and more effective vector control methods for emergencies. Although lyophilized YF vaccine is stable at ambient environmental temperatures, immune responses lower than the expected 95% have been reported in recent mass campaigns, underscoring the need to ensure the proper storage and use of reconstituted vaccine. Modifications to improve the stability of reconstituted vaccine would facilitate vaccine implementation in the field.

7. Status of elimination/eradication efforts to date

The inclusion of YF vaccine in the national EPI has been reported, at one time or another, in only 17 of the 34 at-risk African countries and, except for Gambia, coverage rates have ranged from <1% to 55%. Nigeria, the site of the largest outbreaks in recent times, has a coverage rate <1%. In June 1997, the Executive Committee of the Directing Council of PAHO adopted a resolution urging Member States to include yellow fever vaccine in their national immunization programmes in all areas at risk of transmission of the virus. Five countries in the Americas (Brazil, French Guiana, Panama, Peru, and Trinidad and Tobago) have included the vaccine in the EPI in specified high-risk areas, and others have been encouraged to follow suit.

8. Principal challenges to elimination/eradication

Although a safe and effective YF vaccine has been available for more than 50 years, the failure to control yellow fever in Africa is due to failure of effective application. Although WHO and UNICEF agreed in 1988 that YF vaccine should be included in the EPI of African countries, implementation of that recommendation has been slow and incomplete. The Global Programme on Vaccines strategic plan outlines needed actions for successful implementation of childhood vaccines, citing the specific roles of national governments, international organizations, the donor assistance community and industry. Those parties should collaborate to examine the obstacles that slowed the implementation plan and to improve its performance within a specified period of time. A similar but more selective initiative is needed in South America.

Workgroup participants

1. Sustainable Health and Development Workgroup

Barbiero, Victor	USAID
Bell, Peter	CARE
Broun, Denis	UNICEF
Brown, Peter	Emory University
Daulaire, Nils	USAID
Foster, Stan	Rollins School of Public Health
Garrett, Dwayne	Lions Clubs International
Henderson, Ralph	WHO
Homeida, Mamoun	Higher National Committee for the Control of Onchocerciasis
Jarrett, Stephen	UNICEF PLADS, Freeport
Justice, Judith	University of California, San Francisco
Kotz, Renee	American Red Cross
Kreysler, Joachim	International Federation of Red Cross and Red Crescent Societies
Lawrence, Robert	Johns Hopkins University
Malison, Michael	CDC
Melgaard, Bjorn	WHO
Middleberg, Maurice	CARE
Minkin, Stephen	UNDP
Newberry, David	CARE
O'Rourke, Pearl	NIH
Rodriquez-Garcia, Rosalia	George Washington University
Rojanapitthayakor, Wiwat	Ministry of Public Health, Thailand
Salisbury, David	Department of Health, United Kingdom
Scott, Linda	NIH
Sencer, David	CDC (ret.)
Sergeant, William	The Rotary Foundation
Steinglass, Robert	BASICS
Stokes, Charlie	CDC Foundation
Wahlstrom, Margareta	International Federation of Red Cross and Red Crescent Societies
Waldman, Ron	BASICS
White, Mark	CDC
Widdus, Roy	WHO

2. Noninfectious Diseases Workgroup

Alnwick, David	UNICEF
Baldwin, Bob	CDC
Beresford, Shirley	University of Washington
Blount, Steve	CDC
Corber, Stephen	PAHO
Curran, James	Emory University
Dayrit, Manuel	Aetna HealthCare, Inc.
DeLange, Francois	ICCIDD
Freire, Wilma	PAHO
Hahn, Robert	CDC
Hall, Robert	South Australian Health Commission
Heywood, Peter	The World Bank
Johnston, Richard	March of Dimes
Katz, Martha	CDC Foundation
Kavishe, Festo	UNICEF
Lyerla, Rob	CDC
Maberly, Glen	Rollins School of Public Health
Malaspina, Alex	ILSI
Mannar, M.G.	The Micronutrient Initiative/RC
Marks, James	CDC

Martorell, Reynaldo	Rollins School of Public Health
Mbidde, Edward	Uganda-CWRU Research Colloraboration
Oakley, Godfrey	CDC
Orinda, Vincent	UNICEF
Sommer, Alfred	Johns Hopkins University
Teutsch, Steven	Merck & Co.
Trowbridge, Fredrick	ILSI
Underwood, Barbara	National Eye Institute
Young, Mary Eming	The World Bank

3. Bacterial Diseases Workgroup

Arita, Isao	Agency for Cooperation in International Health
Bart, Kenneth	San Diego State University
Bennett, John	Rollins School of Public Health, Emory University
Berkelman, Ruth	CDC
Berkley, Seth	The International AIDS Vaccine Initiative
Broome, Claire	CDC
Brunham, Robert	University of Manitoba
Cardenas, Carlos	CARE
Castro, Kenneth	CDC
Cook, Joseph	The Edna McConnell Clark Foundation
Counts, George	NIH
Enarson, Donald	International Union Against TB & Lung Disease
Fishbein, Martin	Annenburg School of Communication
Gangarosa, Eugene	Emory University
Garnett, Geoffrey	Oxford University
Gunawan, Suriadi	National Institute on Health Research & Development
Haddix, Anne	CDC
Hierholzer, Walter	CDC
Hinman, Alan	The Task Force for Child Survival and Development
Hughes, James	CDC
Levine, Myron	University of Maryland School of Medicine
Levine, William	CDC
Madore, Dace	Wyeth-Lederle Vaccines and Pediatrics
Makela, Helena	National Public Health Institute
Novotny, Thomas	The World Bank
Nunn, P.P.	WHO
Osterholm, Michael	Minnesota Department of Health
Ostroff, Stephen	CDC
Reingold, Arthur	University of California at Berkeley
Spiegel, Rick	CDC
Stoeckel, Philippe	Association pour L'Aide à la Médicine Préventive
Suskind, Robert M.	International Centre for Diarrhoeal Disease Research, Dhaka, Bangladesh
Valdiserri, Ronald	CDC
Wasserheit, Judith	CDC

4. Parasitic Diseases Workgroup

Acharya, Arnab	Harvard Center for Population and Development Studies

Addiss, David	CDC
Agle, Andrew	The Carter Center
Arias, Jorge	PAHO/WHO
Baraka, Omer	Institute of Endemic Diseases, University of Khartoum, Sudan
Behbehani, Kazem	WHO
Breman, Joel	The Fogarty International Center, NIH
Colley, Daniel	CDC
Coyne, Philip	Food and Drug Administration
Dias, Joao Carlos	Oswaldo Cruz Foundation
Dreyer, Gerusa	Oswaldo Cruz Foundation
El Hassan, Ahmed	University of Copenhagen
Figueroa, Peter	Jamaica Ministry of Health
Gachuhi, Kimani	KEMRI
Guderian, Ronald	Catholic University of Guayaquil, Hospital Vozandes
Hopkins, Donald	The Carter Center
Kappus, Karl	CDC
Karam, Marc	WHO
Lammie, Patrick	CDC
Kurniawan, Agnes	Department of Parasitology, University of Indonesia, Jakarta, Indonesia
McGovern, Victoria	Burroughs Wellcome Fund
Medley, Graham	University of Warwick
Meredith, Stefanie	The Task Force for Child Survival and Development
Miri, Emmanuel	Global 2000
Narayanan, P.R.	Tuberculosis Research Centre
Ndiaye, Jean-Michel	UNICEF
Ndumbe, Peter	University of Yaoundé, Cameroon
Ottesen, Eric	WHO
Packard, Randall	Emory University
Remme, Hans	WHO
Richards, Frank	The Carter Center
Ruiz, Ernesto	CDC
Sauerbrey, Mauricio	Onchocerciasis Elimination Program of the Americas
Schantz, Peter	CDC
Withers, Craig	Global 2000, The Carter Center
Woolery, Chuck	NCIH
Zingeser, James	The Carter Center
Zucker, Jane	UNICEF

5. Viral Diseases Workgroup

Barreto, Luis	Pasteur Merieux Connaught
Bhamarapravati, Natth	Mahidol University, Bangkok, Thailand
Brandling-Bennett, David	PAHO
Cochi, Stephen	CDC
Coulibaly, Issa Malick	National AIDS/STD/TB Program, Côte d'Ivoire
de Quadros, Ciro	PAHO
Drozdov, Sergey	Academy of Medical Science
Fenner, Frank	The Australian National University
Gilchrist, Shawn	Pasteur Merieux Connaught
Henderson, Donald A.	Johns Hopkins University
Holtgrave, David	CDC
Hull, Harry	WHO
Huynh, Lien Phuong	National Institute of Hygiene and Epidemiology
Jamison, Dean	The World Bank
John, Jacob	Christian Medical College Hospital, Vellore, India
Kassim, Sidibe	CDC/HIV, Côte d'Ivoire
Kostermans, Kees	The World Bank
Losos, Joseph	Health Canada
Mahy, Brian	CDC
McKaig, Cat	CARE
Meegan, James	NIAID, NIH
Okwo, Bele	WHO
Olive, J.M.	WHO
Orenstein, Walter	CDC
Reef, Susan	CDC
Robbins, Fred	Case Western University
Rodier, Guenael	WHO
Russell, Philip	Johns Hopkins University
Sakai, Suomi	UNICEF
Schreuder, Bert	Dutch Ministry of Development Co-operation
Sepulveda, Jaime	National Institute of Public Health
Sutter, Roland	CDC
Vernon, Thomas	Merck & Co. Inc.
Wang, Ke-an	Chinese Academy of Preventive Medicine

Annex C

Co-sponsoring organizations

Burroughs Wellcome Fund
CARE
The Carter Center of Emory University
Centers for Disease Control and Prevention
CDC Foundation
Children's Vaccine Initiative
The Edna McConnell Clark Foundation
GlaxoWellcome
International Life Sciences Institute
International Union of Microbiological Societies
Merck Vaccine Division
National Council for International Health
National Institutes of Health/National Institute of
   Allergy and Infectious Diseases

The Fogarty International Center
Pan American Health Organization
Pasteur, Mérieux, Connaught, USA
The Rockefeller Foundation
Rollins School of Public Health of Emory University
The Task Force for Child Survival and Development
United Nations Children's Fund
United Nations Development Programme
The World Bank
World Federation of Public Health Associations
World Health Organization
Wyeth-Lederle Vaccines and Pediatrics